Creative Therapy in Challenging Situations

Creative Therapy in Challenging Situations introduces readers to the innovative approaches that therapists sometimes take when standardized, paint-by-the-numbers routines don't work. Each chapter presents the story of one or more difficult psychotherapy situations followed by the therapists' descriptions of what they did and why, as well as the outcome that resulted. The authors and their stories span a wide variety of theoretical approaches and contexts, showing how clinicians can improvise beyond everyday scenarios and techniques. This collection of provocative, instructive vignettes from well-known practitioners often generates *"You said what?!"* reactions while encouraging readers to think creatively in the moment in order to reach healthy, innovative outcomes from the trickiest and most unexpected therapeutic scenarios.

Michael F. Hoyt, Ph.D., is a psychologist based in Mill Valley, California. He is the author/editor of numerous publications, including *Single-Session Therapy by Walk-In or Appointment*; *Brief Therapy and Beyond*; and *Therapist Stories of Inspiration, Passion, and Renewal.*

Monte Bobele, Ph.D., is Professor Emeritus of Psychology at Our Lady of the Lake University in San Antonio, Texas. He is the co-editor of *Single-Session Therapy by Walk-In or Appointment* and *When One Hour is All You Have*, and the author of numerous other publications.

Creative Therapy in Challenging Situations

Unusual Interventions to Help Clients

Edited by
Michael F. Hoyt and Monte Bobele

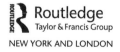

Routledge
Taylor & Francis Group

NEW YORK AND LONDON

First published 2019
by Routledge
52 Vanderbilt Avenue, New York, NY 10017

and by Routledge
2 Park Square, Milton Park, Abingdon, Oxon, OX14 4RN

Routledge is an imprint of the Taylor & Francis Group, an informa business

Library of Congress Cataloging-in-Publication Data
Names: Hoyt, Michael F., editor. | Bobele, Monte, editor.
Title: Creative therapy in challenging situations: unusual interventions to help clients/edited by Michael F. Hoyt & Monte Bobele.
Description: New York, NY: Routledge, 2019. | Includes bibliographical references and index.
Identifiers: LCCN 2018057793 (print) | LCCN 2018058921 (ebook) |
ISBN 9780429028687 (eBook) | ISBN 9780367138097 (hbk) |
ISBN 9780367138103 (pbk) | ISBN 9780429028687 (ebk)
Subjects: | MESH: Psychotherapy–methods | Creativity | Treatment Outcome | Professional-Patient Relations
Classification: LCC RC480.5 (ebook) | LCC RC480.5 (print) | NLM WM 420 |
DDC 616.89/14–dc23
LC record available at https://lccn.loc.gov/2018057793

ISBN: 978-0-367-13809-7 (hbk)
ISBN: 978-0-367-13810-3 (pbk)
ISBN: 978-0-429-02868-7 (ebk)

Typeset in Minion
by Deanta Global Publishing Services, Chennai, India

Dedications
MFH: to Carol Erickson, John Frykman, and Murray Korngold – dear
departed friends and *You Said What?!* aficionados
MB: to Harry Goolishian, John Weakland, and Glen Gardner – who left us all
too early and inspired many *You Said What?!* moments

Contents

Acknowledgments

We express our deep appreciation:

- to the clients whose stories are contained herein and to the authors who wrote the chapters;
- to Lillian Rand and Nina Guttapalle and the editorial board at Routledge Publishers for embracing this project; to Deanta Global Publishing Services for its excellent production; and to all the people whose labor (printing, marketing, sales and delivery, and others) have made it possible;
- to the writers and publishers who permitted use of copyrighted materials;
- to our respective academic and clinical institutions:
  - for Hoyt, Kaiser Permanente and the Stanley Garfield Memorial Award for Clinical Innovation, and the American Psychological Foundation and Nicholas and Dorothy Cummings Foundation for the APF Cummings Psyche Prize;
  - for Bobele, Our Lady of the Lake University San Antonio, Texas and the Houston Galveston Institute, Houston, Texas;
- to our teachers, students, clients, and colleagues;
- to our mentors:
  - for Bobele, Harold Goolishian, Harlene Anderson, George Pulliam, Paul Dell;

- for Hoyt, Jerome L. Singer, Irving Janis, Carl Whitaker, and Bob and Mary Goulding;
- to one another;
- to our friends and families for their love and support.

Michael F. Hoyt, Mill Valley, California
Monte Bobele, San Antonio, Texas

About the Contributors

Editors

Michael F. Hoyt, Ph.D. is a psychologist based in Mill Valley, CA. He was a staff member at Kaiser Permanente for more than 30 years and is a recipient of the APF Cummings Psyche Prize for lifetime contributions to the role of psychologists in organized healthcare. He has been honored as a Continuing Education Distinguished Speaker by both the American Psychological Association and the International Association of Marriage and Family Counselors, and as a Contributor of Note by the Milton H. Erickson Foundation. He has authored and edited numerous books, including *Brief Therapy and Managed Care, Some Stories are Better than Others, The Handbook of Constructive Therapies, Brief Psychotherapies: Principles and Practices, Therapist Stories of Inspiration, Passion, and Renewal: What's Love Got to Do with It?, Capturing the Moment: Single-Session Therapy and Walk-In Services* (with Moshe Talmon), *Single-Session Therapy by Walk-In or Appointment* (with Bobele, Slive, Young, and Talmon), and *Brief Therapy and Beyond: Stories, Language, Love, Hope, and Time.*

Monte Bobele, Ph.D., ABPP is Emeritus Professor of Psychology at Our Lady of the Lake University in San Antonio, Texas and Faculty of the Houston Galveston Institute in Houston, Texas. He is a licensed psychologist and an AAMFT Clinical Fellow and Approved Supervisor. He coedited (with Arnold Slive) *When One Hour is All You Have: Effective Therapy for Walk-In Clients*; he is also coeditor (with Hoyt, Slive, Young, and Talmon) of *Single-Session Therapy by Walk-In or Appointment.* In 2011 he was awarded a Fulbright Specialist Grant to help develop a walk-in service in a university clinic in Mexico City; he has since consulted on the opening of two other walk-in clinics in Mexico, and has taught graduate courses in single-session therapy in the US, Canada, Mexico, and Australia. He has also been involved in programs designed to train culturally and linguistically competent psychologists to work with Spanish-speaking populations and has co-led several immersion programs in Mexico. He was the recipient of the Texas Psychological Association's 2012 Outstanding Contribution to Education Award, and OLLU's 2013 Fleming Award for Teaching Excellence.

Additional Authors

Andrew T. Austin, based in Rustington, West Sussex, England is a leading NLP practitioner and registered nurse. He is the author of *The Rainbow Machine: Tales from a Neurolinguist's Journal.*

Bob Bertolino, Ph.D., based in St. Louis, Missouri, is the author of many books, including *Strengths-Based Engagement and Practice, Therapy on the Front Line*, and *Collaborative, Competency-Based Counseling and Therapy.*

Flavio Cannistrá, Psy.D. is a licensed psychologist based in Rome, Italy. He is the Director of the Italian Center for Single-Session Therapy (Rome) and coeditor (with F. Piccirilli) of *Terapia a Seduta Singola: Principi e Pratiche (Single-Session Therapy: Principles and Practices)*

Jim Duvall, M.Ed., based on Galveston Island, Texas, is a marriage and family therapist and narrative therapy trainer. He is the editor of the *Journal of Systemic Therapies* and coauthor (with L. Béres) of *Innovations in Narrative Therapy: Connecting Practice, Training, and Research.*

Douglas Flemons, Ph.D. is Professor of Family Therapy at Nova Southeastern University in Fort Lauderdale, Florida and author of several books, including *Relational Suicide Assessment* and *Of One Mind: The Logic of Hypnosis, the Practice of Therapy;* and coeditor (with Shelley Green) of *Quickies: The Handbook of Brief Sex Therapy.*

Joseph A. Goldfield, M.S.W., based in New York City, is a psychiatric social worker in private practice. He is the author of various chapters and coeditor (with Judah Ronch) of *Mental Wellness in Aging: Strengths-Based Approaches.*

Shelley Green, Ph.D. is Professor of Family Therapy at Nova Southeastern University in Fort Lauderdale, Florida. She is the author of various chapters and coeditor (with Douglas Flemons) of *Quickies: The Handbook of Brief Sex Therapy.*

Chris Iveson, B.S. is cofounder of BRIEF (formerly known as Brief Therapy Practice) in London, England. His books include *Whose Life? Community Care for Older People and Their Families, Problem to Solution: Brief Therapy with Individuals and Families, Brief Coaching: A Solution-Focused Approach*, and *Solution-Focused Brief Therapy: 100 Key Points and Techniques.*

Bradford Keeney, Ph.D. is a marriage and family therapist based in New Orleans, Louisiana. He is the author of numerous books, including *The Aesthetics of Change, The Creative Therapist*, and the autobiographical *Shaking Out the Spirits;* he is also the subject of *American Shaman: An Odyssey of Global Healing Traditions* (by Jeffrey Kottler, Jon Carlson, and Brad Keeney). He is also coauthor, with Hillary Keeney, of *Circular Therapeutics, Creative Therapeutic Technique*, and *Sacred Ecstatics.*

Hillary Keeney, Ph.D. is a marriage and family therapist based in New Orleans, Louisiana. She is the coauthor (with Brad Keeney) of *Circular Therapeutics, Creative Therapeutic Technique*, and *Sacred Ecstatics*.

David V. Keith, M.D. is Professor of Psychiatry and Family Medicine and Director of Family Therapy at SUNY Upstate Medical University, Syracuse, New York. He is the author of *Continuing the Experiential Approach of Carl Whitaker: Process, Practice, and Magic*; coauthor (with Gary Connell and Linda Connell) of *Defiance in the Family: Finding Hope in Therapy*; coeditor (with Phoebe Prosky) of *Family Therapy as an Alternative to Medication: An Appraisal of Pharmland*; and subject of *Clinical Dialogues in Family Therapy: Based on the Psychotherapy of Carl Whitaker, M.D. and David Keith, M.D.* (by Howard Denofsky).

Jeffrey Kottler, Ph.D. is Adjunct Professor at Baylor College of Medicine in Houston, Texas. He is the author of more than 80 books, including *On Being a Therapist, Creative Breakthroughs in Therapy, Duped: Lies and Deception in Therapy*, and *Their Finest Hour*.

Esther Krohner, M.S., LMFT is a lead therapist at the Brief Therapy Center of the Mental Research Institute in Palo Alto, California; and is also a lead therapist for Bay Area Clinical Associates in Oakland, CA.

Michele Ritterman, Ph.D. is a licensed psychologist based in Berkeley, California. She is the author of *Using Hypnosis in Family Therapy, Hope Under Siege: Terror and Family Support in Chile*, and *The Tao of a Woman: 100 Ways to Turn*.

Karin Schlanger, M.S., LMFT is the Director of Brief Therapy at the Mental Research Institute in Palo Alto, California. She is the coauthor (with Richard Fisch) of *Brief Therapy with Intimidating Cases*, and the coeditor (with Wendel Ray and Richard Fisch) of *Focused Problem Resolution: Selected Papers of the MRI Brief Therapy Center*.

Clara Haydee Solís Ponce, M.S., is Professor of Psychology at the Autonomous University of Mexico (UNAM), Zaragoza campus, Mexico City.

Terry Soo-Hoo, Ph.D. is Professor of Educational Psychology, California State University East Bay, Hayward, California. The author of numerous chapters, he is also the Clinical Director of the Mental Research Institute in Palo Alto, CA.

Pedro Vargas Avalos, M.S. is Professor of Psychology at the Autonomous University of Mexico (UNAM), Zaragoza campus, Mexico City.

"You can't depend on your eyes when your imagination is out of focus."
—Mark Twain

CHAPTER 1

"You Said *What?*"

Introduction and Invitation

Michael F. Hoyt and Monte Bobele

When therapists get together, they often talk about the strange and unusual things that clinicians sometimes do to help clients. The stories are always interesting and provocative and often instructive. Several times we have heard someone say, "You said *what?*" and "Gosh, that ought to be in a book – I'd buy and read it!" *Creative Therapy in Challenging Situations: Unusual Interventions to Help Clients* aims to address that need.

The main objective of this book is to illustrate, with modern examples, ways therapists can work creativity, effectively, and ethically in challenging situations to help clients expand options and embrace healthy choices.[1] Clinicians often wonder, "What should I do?" when, confronted with complex circumstances, standardized, paint-by-the-numbers routines aren't likely to work or are just plain boring. Our purpose is to encourage readers to embrace artistry and originality ("think outside the box") and to offer some specific intervention examples for those struggling with the sometimes-daunting tasks of assisting troubled and troubling clients.

Getting Inspired

During our training and many years of practice, we have been influenced by the wizardry of Milton Erickson, the strategic therapy maneuvers of Jay Haley and Cloé Madanes, the conjuring magic of Carl Whitaker, the many brilliant gambits of the MRI crew, the penetrating family therapy of Salvador Minuchin, the provocative therapy of Frank Farrelly and Jeff Brandsma, the subtlety of Harry Goolishian, the "reverse psychology" of paradoxical psychotherapy, the innovations of the Milan school of family therapy, and other unconventional approaches[2].

Invitation to Authors

With these pioneering therapists' creative inspirations percolating in our heads, we sent the following invitation to some leading clinician-colleagues:

CREATIVE THERAPY IN CHALLENGING SITUATIONS: YOU SAID WHAT?

Dear Colleague,

We are writing to invite you to contribute to a new and unusual book, one that discusses the counterintuitive, surprising, seemingly strange, and occasionally shocking things that therapists sometimes do to help clients. We have all heard about (and have sometimes done) unusual things in therapy. Consider these examples from the lore and literature:

- A highly anxious client who has panic attacks is asked to bring on panic during the session.
- A sex therapist prohibits a couple from having intercourse despite prescribing arousing exercises.
- A client seeking help for nocturnal enuresis is instructed to urinate into the bed before getting in at night.
- A quarreling couple is encouraged to pick a fight with one another when they are not mad.
- A psychiatric hospital patient who claims to be Jesus Christ is put to work in the carpenter shop.
- A prideful stroke-victim who has fallen into a deep funk is provoked with humiliating taunts.
- The therapist of another stroke victim throws himself on the floor and asks the patient to teach him how to get up.
- A therapist invites his lonely patient to be his doubles partner at the tennis club they both belong to.
- A woman with a pathologically jealous boyfriend is told "You may have to stand in front of his loaded gun and let him pull the trigger so that he will understand that you love him so much you would be willing to give up your life to prove your love for him."
- A teenage girl is in the E.R. after taking a little overdose to spite the boyfriend who had just dumped her. The consulting psychiatrist asks a series of questions, like if she were dead who would get her favorite hairbrush, who would get her clothes, how long does she think it would take before the ex-boyfriend was dating someone else, etc.
- A paranoid, vengeful patient is told that he can make the persons he is angry at suffer more by leaving them in terror than by attacking them.
- A woman who reports always thinking about suicide is advised to carry a vial of poison in her purse.

We are interested in assembling a collection of case vignettes that illustrate how and when (and when not) to use unusual, sometimes risky or perilous interventions. We are looking for reports with the following characteristics:

- well written (give it an interesting title and use an engaging style), appropriately disguised to protect client privacy/confidentiality;
- illustrating an unusual intervention that occurred in a "high-risk" (e.g., suicide/homicide, abuse, psychosis, intoxication/addiction, majorly distressed relationship) situation;
- with a discussion of context—situation, problem, participants; what was done (perhaps including some dialogue), why you thought it would work, what resulted; and what principles could be garnered for use by other clinicians, including cultural nuances, theoretical explanations, and any cautions (including ethical considerations) you might suggest about when *not* to do something similar

The response was enthusiastic. Each contributor is an active practitioner, a frequent workshop presenter, or university professor. Some are former students or colleagues of the well-known therapists cited earlier. All are skillful writers, having published books, chapters, and articles. They identify with diverse theoretical orientations:

- *Strategic-interactional therapy influenced by the seminal work at the Mental Research Institute* – Bobele in Chapter 4, Shelley Green in Chapter 9, Hoyt in Chapter 10, Karin Schlanger and Esther Krohner in Chapter 17, Clara Solís and Pedro Vargas in Chapter 18, and Terry Soo-Hoo in Chapter 19;
- *Ericksonian-inspired therapy* – Andy Austin in Chapter 2, Douglas Flemons in Chapter 7, Hoyt in Chapter 11, and Michele Ritterman in Chapter 16;
- *Solution-focused/solution-oriented therapy* – Bob Bertolino in Chapter 3 and Chris Iveson in Chapter 12;
- *Narrative therapy* – Jim Duvall in Chapter 6;
- *Improvisational therapy and circular therapeutics* – Hillary and Brad Keeney in Chapter 13;
- *Symbolic experiential therapy* – David Keith in Chapter 14;
- *Eclectic/integrative and harder-to-categorize therapies* – including Flavio Cannistrá in Chapter 5, Joe Goldfield in Chapter 8, and Jeffrey Kottler in Chapter 15.[3]

Each chapter contains a brief description of one or more challenging situations, what the therapist did and why, what resulted, and a discussion of issues that were considered. All cases were conducted in English, unless otherwise noted; all have been appropriately disguised to protect clients'[4] confidentiality. This collection represents a wide range of approaches. Chapters are arranged alphabetically by author's last name. We hope the chapters will stimulate new ways of thinking and may suggest some interventions that can be adapted to different clinical contexts. The book is intended for practicing mental-health professionals and graduate students. It will have special appeal to those who identify with "brief therapy," of course – that is, Ericksonians, MRI strategic therapists, NLPers, solution-focused and narrative therapists, and their kin – as well as others who are interested in expanding their skill sets.

Playing for Real

Gregory Bateson (1953/1972, p. 14) began one of his "metalogues" with the following imaginary conversation:

Daughter: Daddy, are these conversations serious?

Father: Certainly they are.

Daughter: They're not a sort of game you play with me?

Father: God forbid … but they are a sort of game we play together.

Daughter: Then they're *not* serious!

We also recall that Paul Watzlawick (1983) entitled one of his books *The Situation Is Hopeless but Not Serious*, and elsewhere (1978, p. 119) wrote: "Let us remember: We never deal with reality *per se*, but rather with *images* of reality – that is with interpretations." Cloé Madanes (2006, p. 33) averred: "And most of all, you must love to provide the spark that bridges the gap between limitations and possibilities, knowing that there's a great deal to human beings, so a great deal can be made out of them. They don't have to stay the way they are now, and we don't have to see them only as they are now, but also as they might become." This spirit, we think, also informed the advice given by Milton Erickson (1954, p. 127): "Emphasis should be placed more upon what the patient does in the present and will do in the future than upon a mere understanding of why some long-past event occurred."

They were all pointing, as do the authors in this book, to the importance of building one's sense of reality with a spirit of play and creativity.

And Now …

At a time when our field is in danger of being dominated by oversold manualized protocols (see Leichsenring et al., 2018) and excessive psychopharmacology (see Hoyt & Gurman, 2012/2017), we hope you will find in the chapters that follow a range of innovative ideas, interventions, and inspirations. After the contributing authors present their various stories, we will provide an Editors' Conclusion that gleans ideas and offers some lessons to be learned.

Notes

1 This volume arose partly out of discussions we had in a previous collaboration (Hoyt, Bobele, Slive, Young, & Talmon, 2018). As we talked about interventions in

risky situations, we realized that there are many interesting examples – and this book was conceived.

2 A partial reading list would include Andreas (2006); Battino (2015); Bergman (1985); Boscolo, Cecchin, Hoffman, & Penn (1987); Corsini (2001); Cummings and Sayama (1995); de Shazer (1982); Dolan (1985); Erickson (1980); Farrelly and Brandsma (1974); Fisch and Schlanger (1999); Fisch, Weakland, and Segal (1982); Haley (1963, 1973, 1977, 1984, 1985; Haley and Richeport-Haley (1993); Hoyt (1994, 1996, 1998); Keeney (1991); Kottler and Carlson (2008, 2009); Loriedo and Vella, 1992; Madanes (1981, 1984, 1990, 2006); Minuchin (1974; Minuchin & Fishman, 1981; Minuchin & Reiter, 2013); O'Hanlon (1999; O'Hanlon & Hexum, 1990); Neill and Kniskern (1982); Pittman (1984); Rosen (1982); Selvini Palazzoli, Cecchin, Prata, and Boscolo (1978); Watzlawick, Weakland, and Fisch, (1974); Weeks (1991; Weeks & L'Abate, 1982); and Whitaker and Ryan (1989).

3 A *You Said What?* intervention doesn't necessarily have to be drawn from the world of Brief Therapy, either. One of us (MFH, 1974 in Madison, Wisconsin) had a memorable *You Said What?* experience when he saw the noted psychoanalyst Harold Searles (see Searles, 1965) say to a glowering, regressed psychotic patient, "You just threw acid in my face" and the patient said "No, I didn't" and Searles replied, "Then what was it?" For a discussion of Georg Groddeck, who was called "The Wild Analyst," see Grossman and Grossman (1965); for a review of the controversies involving John Rosen's "Direct Analysis," see Balbuena (2015).

4 Throughout the volume, the term *client* (rather than *patient*) is preferred. The former appellation emphasizes competence and an egalitarian connection whereas the latter tends to evoke images of pathology and dependency (see Hoyt, 2017, pp. 217–218).

References

Andreas, S. (2006). *Six blind elephants: Understanding ourselves and each other* (Vols. 1 & 2). Moab, UT: Real People Press.

Balbuena, F. (2015). Revisiting Dr. Rosen: Villain or unjustly treated innovator? *International Forum of Psychoanalysis, 24*(3), 172–181.

Bateson, G. (1972). Metalogue: About games and being serious. In *Steps to ecology of mind* (pp. 14–20). New York: Ballantine Books. (work originally published 1953).

Battino, R. (2015). *When all else fails: Some new and some old tools for doing brief therapy.* Bethel, CT: Crown House Publishing.

Bergman, J.S. (1985). *Fishing for barracuda: Pragmatics of brief systemic therapy.* New York: Norton.

Boscolo, L., Cecchin, G., Hoffman, L., & Penn, P. (1987). *Milan systemic family therapy: Conversations in theory and practice.* New York: Basic Books.

Corsini, R.J. (Ed.) (2001). *Handbook of innovative therapy* (2nd ed.). New York: Wiley.

Cummings, N. & Sayama, M. (1995). *Focused psychotherapy: A casebook of brief, intermittent psychotherapy through the life cycle.* New York: Routledge.

de Shazer, S. (1982). *Patterns of brief family therapy.* New York: Guilford Press.

Dolan, Y.M. (1985). *A path with a heart: Ericksonian utilization with resistant and chronic clients.* New York: Brunner/Mazel.

Erickson, M.H. (1954). Special techniques of brief psychotherapy. *Journal of Clinical and Experimental Hypnosis, 2,* 109–129.

Erickson, M.H. (1980). *Collected papers* (Vols. 1–4; E.L. Rossi, Ed.). New York: Irvington.

Farrelly, F. & Brandsma, J. (1974). *Provocative therapy*. Capitola, CA: Meta Publications.

Fisch, R., & Schlanger, K. (1999). *Brief therapy with intimidating cases: Changing the unchangeable*. San Francisco: Jossey-Bass.

Fisch, R., Weakland, J.H., & Segal, L. (1982). *The tactics of change: Doing therapy briefly*. San Francisco: Jossey-Bass.

Grossman, C.M., & Grossman, S. (1965). *The wild analyst: The life and work of Georg Groddeck*. New York: Braziller.

Haley, J. (1963). *Strategies of psychotherapy*. New York: Grune & Stratton.

Haley, J. (1973). *Uncommon therapy: The psychiatric techniques of Milton H. Erikson, M.D.* New York: Norton.

Haley, J. (1977). *Problem-solving therapy: New strategies for effective family therapy*. San Francisco: Jossey-Bass.

Haley, J. (1984). *Ordeal therapy: Unusual ways to change behavior*. San Francisco: Jossey-Bass.

Haley, J. (1985). *Conversations with Milton H. Erickson, M.D.* (Vols. 1–3). New York: Triangle Press.

Hoyt, M.F. (Ed.). (1994). *Constructive therapies*. New York: Guilford Press.

Hoyt, M.F. (Ed.). (1996). *Constructive therapies 2*. New York: Guilford Press.

Hoyt, M.F. (Ed.). (1998). *The handbook of constructive therapies: Innovative approaches from leading practitioners*. San Francisco: Jossey-Bass.

Hoyt, M.F. (2017). *Brief therapy and beyond: Stories, language, love, hope, and time*. New York: Routledge.

Hoyt, M.F., & Gurman, A.S. (2012). Wither couple/family therapy? *The Family Journal: Counseling and Therapy for Couples and Families*, 20(1), 13–17. Reprinted in M.F. Hoyt, *Brief therapy and beyond: Stories, language, love, hope, and time* (pp. 287–293). New York: Routledge, 2017.

Hoyt, M. F., & Richeport, M. (1993). *Milton H. Erickson, M. D.: Explorer in hypnosis and therapy*. [Videotape/DVD]. New York: Brunner-Mazel.

Keeney, B. P. (1991). *Improvisational therapy: A practical guide for creative clinical strategies*. New York: Guilford Press.

Kottler, J., & Carlson, J. (2008). *Their finest hour: Master therapists share their greatest success stories*. Bethel, CT: Crown House Publishers.

Kottler, J., & Carlson, J. (2009). *Creative breakthroughs in therapy: Tales of transformation and astonishment*. New York: Wiley.

Leichsenring, F., Abbass, A., Hilsenroth, M.J., Luyten, P., Munder, T., Rabung, S., & Steinert, C. (2018). "Gold standards," plurality and monocultures: The need for diversity in psychotherapy. *Frontiers in Psychiatry, 24*, April. https://doi.org/10.3389/fpsyt.2018.00157.

Loriedo, C., & Vella, G. (1992). *Paradox and the family system*. New York: Brunner/Mazel.

Madanes, C. (1981). *Strategic family therapy*. San Francisco: Jossey-Bass.

Madanes, C. (1984). *Behind the one-way mirror: Advances in the practice of strategic therapy*. San Francisco: Jossey-Bass.

Madanes, C. (1990). *Sex, love, and violence: Strategies for transformation*. New York: Norton.

Madanes, C. (2006). Remembering our heritage. In *The therapist as humanist, social activist, and systemic thinker ... and other selected papers* (pp. 24–33). Phoenix, AZ: Zeig, Tucker, & Theisen.

Minuchin, S. (1974). *Families and family therapy*. Cambridge, MA: Harvard University Press.

Minuchin, S., & Fishman, H.C. (1981). *Family therapy techniques*. Cambridge, MA: Harvard University Press.

Minuchin, S., & Reiter, M.D. (2013). *The craft of family therapy: Challenging certainties*. New York: Routledge.

Neill, J.R., & Kniskern, D.P. (Eds.). (1982). *From psyche to system: The evolving therapy of Carl Whitaker*. New York: Guilford Press.

O'Hanlon, W.H. (1999). *Do one thing different: And other uncommonly sensible solutions to life's persistent problems*. New York: William Morrow.

O'Hanlon, W.H., & Hexum, A.L. (1990). *An uncommon casebook: The complete clinical work of Milton H. Erickson, M.D.* New York: Norton.

Pittman, F.S., III. (1984). Wet Cocker Spaniel therapy: An essay on technique in family therapy. *Family Process, 23*, 1–9.

Rosen, S. (1982). *My voice will go with you: The teaching tales of Milton H. Erickson*. New York: Norton.

Selvini Palazzoli, M. S., Boscolo, L. Cecchin, G., & Prata, G. (1978). *Paradox and counterparadox*. New York: Jason Aronson.

Searles, H.F. (1965). *Collected papers on schizophrenia and related subjects*. New York: International Universities Press.

Watzlawick, P. (1978). *The language of change: Elements of therapeutic communication*. New York: Norton.

Watzlawick, P. (1983). *The situation is hopeless, but not serious*. New York: Dutton.

Watzlawick, P., Weakland, J.H., & Fisch, R. (1974). *Change: Principles of problem formation and problem resolution*. New York: Norton.

Weeks, G.R. (Ed.) (1991). *Promoting change through paradoxical therapy*. New York: Brunner/Mazel.

Weeks, G.R., & L'Abate, L. (1982). *Paradoxical psychotherapy: Theory and practice with individuals, couples, and families*. New York: Brunner/Mazel.

Whitaker, C., & Ryan, M. O. (1989). *Midnight musings of a family therapist*. New York: Norton.

CHAPTER 2

The Accidental Drug Dealer

Andrew T. Austin

Sarah presented a problem that is just all too common – cocaine addiction. But it came with a number of added complications. The background story was a little like this. Married, children, successful, wealthy, she and her husband like to entertain guests at dinner parties.

Children sent to bed, wine opened, conversations and gossip, neighborhood scandal and talk of business success. This became a regular Friday night thing.

Then one evening a guest suggested they all try cocaine, which, it just so happened, he had brought along with him. And in that moment, "Everything changed," Sarah told me, "I just loved it, we all did." And from then onwards, a Friday night dinner party was not the same without cocaine.

"Before I knew it I was buying it in bulk," Sarah explained. "Well, it made sense, you see, to buy on behalf of everyone." Yes, dear reader, without really thinking about it, this nice, respectable, upper-middle-class housewife had inadvertently become a drug dealer.

The dinner parties became more popular and extravagant. They went on for longer. Ever bigger sums of money changed hands.

"Sounds great," I told her, before asking, "So what is the problem?"

The problem was that things were clearly getting out of control. "The children are getting older and I worry that they will find out and realize what is going on." Personally, from a child's point of view, I'd have thought this would not be as bad as she might have imagined. After all, if I were regularly sent off to bed so that mum and dad could have yet another "special party" with all their friends, I wouldn't necessarily be assuming it was just drugs.

The other problem was that she really wanted to stop all of this, put an end to it all, get rid of her "useless drug addict friends and all the hangers-on."

"So why don't you?" I asked.

"My husband has no intention of doing any such thing and puts pressure on me to conform to it all," she told me. Sarah went on to explain how guilty she felt because she was the one who had basically driven the entire enterprise at the beginning but now had lost control of it all.

"Sometimes I just pretend to take some, so he and the others don't give me a hard time about not joining in."

It became increasingly clear to me that this was not an issue of addiction, nor was it an issue for one-to-one therapy. When someone feels that they need to pretend to use drugs in order to find social acceptance, there is a much wider systemic issue at play. Regardless, from a therapeutic point of view, it seemed that the issue of the children could be exploited for leverage within this system.

"What about the children?" I asked, "Don't you worry that they might ingest the drugs sometime by accident?"

"No, not at all, we keep the cocaine in a drug cabinet in the bathroom," Sarah assured me and went on to explain. For those who aren't familiar, drug cabinets are bolted to the wall, much like a safe box might be, and are a locked cabinet that, in turn, have another lockable unit inside them. Hospitals use these to store the opioids and other legally classified medications. In turn, the cocaine was kept in clear "bank bags," polythene money bags with sleeve/pockets for additional paperwork.

The self-assuredness with which she explained all this safety concerned me. Sarah's concern clearly was not for the physical safety of her children, but rather was about what her children might think of her should they find out about the cocaine. For her, this was a moral issue, an issue of judgment, not an issue of addiction. This would be easy. I knew what to do.

"Close your eyes," I told her directly. No warm up, no relaxation, just "close your eyes" and I began a simple induction: "Take a deep breath and relax and pay attention carefully to my words."

Something that took me a long time to learn was that induction needs to be proportional to the intervention. Conventional hypnosis looks like this: relax the client deeply and then give suggestions. But I was rarely convinced that this would necessarily be effective. It might be sometimes, but other times the client might just be sitting there conforming to the therapist's wishes, full of doubts about the efficacy and worried if they are going to get their money's worth.

So, I learned that not all trances are the same and neither are all inductions. For example, some hypnotists like to use a shock induction. This rapid induction method works very effectively on the stage and can be utilized for dramatic effect. It usually involves tipping the client backwards off balance and gently easing them to the floor whilst commanding "SLEEP!" to the hapless subject. But, if I use a rapid shock induction, would this induce the type of trance that was useful for my purposes if, for example, my client wished to stop smoking. Maybe instead I could tip them backwards and command, "STOP SMOKING!" as I *lowered* them down?

When working with an anxious client, why put the helpful suggestions inside a nice relaxed trance? Would it not be better to put at least some of the change inside the trance that matches the problem state?

Now, there are some things you need to know. Back in the '90s when I did this session, I had a sizable reputation as an Ericksonian hypnotherapist.[1] I did long fancy inductions, full of clever language patterns, stunning intonations and charm. I was really good at eliciting full hypnotic phenomena; one of my favorites being the bald man to whom I gave the suggestion that he would be able to hear his hair growing. I thought it worth a try, but he was back early the next day after a sleepless night and an itchy head. "It sounds like fucking termites!" were his exact words to me as he entered the doorway. His hair didn't grow, and he wanted his money back, but I guess it was at least worth a try.

So, this cocaine lady was expecting something from me – as with most clients, Sarah was expecting both financial satisfaction and effective remedy of the problem. This is an important aspect of hypnotherapy that ought to be considered more widely.

Hypnotherapy invariably uses a clinical metaphor, that of modern surgery. In modern general surgery there exists the patient and the surgeon. The patient submits themselves to the will and expertise of the surgeon. The patient is not involved in performing the operation and is generally expected to be entirely passive to the situation. So much so that not only is the patient rendered unconscious, but paralyzing agents are administered, too. Surgeons don't like it when their subjects are squirming around and making screaming noises. It ruins the atmosphere and tends to make the operation more difficult, so forced compliance is king. Anesthetics make the whole operation quite painless for the patient. At least that is the plan.

Anyway, this is no different in hypnosis. The patient surrenders to the will of the hypnotist, is usually rendered deeply relaxed or even cataleptic, and when virtually unconscious, the hypnotist goes to work. And when the whole operation is over, the hypnotist wakes up the client who reports back that he remembers little of what the hypnotist said and did. Ideally the whole procedure is quite painless. No participation from the client is needed.

Now let us go back to our cocaine lady. Was the problem her unconscious? I doubted it. Instead Sarah had become the victim of her own success as an accidental drug dealer. It seemed to me that the main problems were her husband's recklessness, his lack of support, her awful friends and her lack of social power to be able to stand firm in the face of these challenges.

All of these problems were extraneous to the relationship between her and me, and none of them resided in her subconscious. In short, this was not a therapeutic issue and yet she brought the issue to a hypnotherapist. This was like making an appointment to see your proctologist to ask him to fix your leaking tap. "Where's the tap?" he asks in bemusement. "Oh, it's back at my house" you tell him. So much therapy actually looks like this to me.

So anyway, back to the protagonist of this story. Although it hadn't been mentioned I thought it might be reasonable for me to assume that all this life drama and emerging crisis was occurring within a trance of disappointment.

Disappointment that her social affairs didn't work the way she had hoped, disappointment in her husband's conduct, disappointment in her friends, disappointment in herself. Most of all though, disappointment that the drug of the hour didn't deliver on its promise of a better life. Just look at how alcoholic drinks are advertised. They don't promote these things with images of domestic and street violence, homelessness, loneliness, liver disease, and social failure. No, they suggest that their beverage will give you a better life. It's the lie of the drug.

So, with this lady, I was going for a trance of disappointment. The Great Ericksonian Hypnotist to whom she had just paid a lot of money shall also fail to deliver upon her expectation in order to create the correct trance into which to send the hypnotic suggestion that I hoped would create a systemic change in her thinking. She was, of course, expecting a long fancy-pants induction, hypnotic phenomena, amnesia, and of course, most important of all, a complete and miraculous cure of her situation. But at this moment in time, she didn't yet know that this was exactly what she wasn't going to get.

So, back to the story. I'd just told her to close her eyes and listen carefully to my words. She did as I instructed.

> I am not going to tell you to change your behavior, in fact, I am going to tell you to continue exactly as you are. Now listen really carefully, I want you to do one thing. Just one thing differently. And I want you to agree to do this thing before I tell you what it is. It will be fine, I want you to do this thing, do you agree?

Sarah nodded agreement.

Now, to interrupt this story again for a moment: what on earth would possess anyone to agree to these terms? What kind of idiot would actually do this? Why would anyone agree to something before they even knew what it was? This was exactly the reason she was in the situation with the cocaine to begin with. She went for it before she stopped to think about what it was she was getting into. This is a common issue with any form of drug use – the sacrifice of the long-term benefits of not having the drug in exchange for the short-term pleasures it offers.

My request to her was the perfect pace and lead, matching her state and situation to increase rapport before offering direction[2]. "Continue exactly as you are," I said, "the only thing I want you to do is…" – and I paused for effect, just a little bit too long in order to create an awkwardness – "Listen, I want you to keep everything the same, I just want you to add a photograph of your children to the bank bags."

And at that her eyes snapped open and she looked at me in horror, "I cannot do that!" she said in a tone of distress. And at that I said, "and now you can leave" in the same hypnotic tone I had been using just before her eyes had opened. I ushered her straight out the door.

It took about ten days before I heard from Sarah again. Actually, I was just leaving the office to go and visit a friend as she was getting out of her car.

"I was just popping by to tell you," she said, "I stood outside for ages wondering whether to come back in after you told me to leave. I didn't know what to do. I got home and told my husband that this stops today, or I'll take the children and leave. He just laughed and tried to make out that I was just being neurotic."

"Then what happened?" I asked.

"I packed my things, took my children and left. The whole time he just watched me, laughing, and saying that it wouldn't be long before I came back. I won't be going back. I've already seen a lawyer to file for divorce."

She came back to see me about three years later to thank me.

"You made me realize what was important. I just hope that one day my ex-husband learns the same."

She was already referring to him as "ex-husband."

So, it's worth a mention of what actually happened here, why such a simple change created such a significant shift in the client's thinking. It was the drug cabinet, you see. This was quite an unusual and really specific thing for any mother to do, and it was anchored to Sarah's sense of self-assuredness. It was this very thing that was stabilizing the system.

The drug cabinet had one specific purpose, which was to separate the world of cocaine from her image as a respectable mother with young children. The drug cabinet did this by acting as a safety barrier between Sarah and her children, not just physically, but also mentally. In addition to its practical use, it also enabled her to mentally compartmentalize her drug life from the children's lives.

Furthermore, it was worth noting that the peer pressure from her social scene and her husband were too great, and certainly exerted a force greater than anything I'd be able to raise myself. What was needed was something no reasonable mother was able to ignore – the love of, and for, her children.

A mother's world of children is full of looking ahead in time, pre-planning, mentally assessing risks, paying close attention to cues and clues. It also involves progressive change and movement through time. It is forward thinking, it is proactive. Meanwhile the world of cocaine is largely reactive and short term, and in her case, it is full of regret and remorse and backward/retrospective thinking. It is passive. So, I'd gotten her to mentally insert a pro-active principle into the center of that backward passive world – the drug cabinet.

From a therapeutic point of view, it was a win–win. Remember, she opened her eyes in protest and said she wouldn't be doing that. Of course, mentally, it had already happened. From within her disappointment trance, she literally stood up for herself for once. She was ushered out the door lest she have time to talk herself around again in her verbal engagements with me.

In her mind, she had separated her children from the world of cocaine. Basically, all I really needed to do was to get her to put a mental picture of her children inside the cocaine world and leave the rest to maternal instinct. It was this maternal instinct that led her to remove herself and her children from such a seedy environment.

Notes

1 For more on Ericksonian hypnosis and neurolinguistic programming, see Austin (2007; www.23NLPeople.com), Bandler and Grinder (1975), and Andreas (2006).
2 "The beginning of this process we call *pacing*.... The hypnotist begins to describe the experiences he knows by observation the client is having.... This is, in fact, equivalent to meeting the client at his model of the world – going to the client's reality, accepting it, and then utilizing it for the purposes of the hypnotic session. Meeting a client at his model of the world, pacing that model and then leading it into new territory is one of Erickson's consistent strategies which make his work easier both for himself and for his client" (Bandler & Grinder, 1975, pp. 137–138).

References

Andreas, S. (2006). *Six blind elephants: Understanding ourselves and each other* (Vols. 1 & 2). Boulder, CO: Real People Press.

Austin, A.T. (2007). *The rainbow machine: Tales from a neurolinguist's journal.* Boulder, CO: Real People Press.

Bandler, R., & Grinder, J. (1975). *Patterns in the hypnotic techniques of Milton H. Erickson, M.D.* (Vol. 1). Cupertino CA: Meta Publications.

CHAPTER 3

A Different Kind of Education

Bob Bertolino

Early in my career, back in the late 1980s, my experience with family therapy was still in its infancy. My subsequent education has involved both the Mental Research Institute (MRI) in Palo Alto, California (Watzlawick, Weakland, & Fisch, 1974) and the "Washington" schools of strategic family therapy (Haley, 1987; Madanes, 1981), as well as studies of solution-focused and solution-oriented therapies, which align well with my "personal philosophy" about the role of people's strengths and abilities in the service of change (Bertolino, 1999; O'Hanlon & Weiner-Davis, 2003). Furthermore, through personal training with Bill O'Hanlon, I have gained a more profound understanding of the influence of the psychiatrist Milton H. Erickson (e.g., see O'Hanlon, 1987; O'Hanlon & Hexum, 1990). As my skills in hypnosis grew, I learned ways of thinking more creatively about clients and their situations. I also found the mid- to late '90s to be a fertile time to learn given the emergence of a new wave of therapies that emphasized strengths, collaboration, and the reauthoring of client narratives (Hoyt, 1994, 1996). I see clients as capable, and view problems as hurdles rather than barriers to their futures.

Early on, what I lacked experience-wise, I made up for with hope. I was "green," as they say, but I understood that hope was not a strategy. Instead, it was what I leaned on when met with situations that I did not yet have a broad enough repertoire of skills to manage, which was often. The one thing I knew was that I would not give up on any of the youth and families I saw for therapy. And I certainly needed hope when I met Laura, Jim, and Keith.

Case Report: "Whatever It Takes"

Laura, a 43-year-old mother of two, called me about her 15-year-old son, Keith. In our brief phone call, she summarized that Keith had been skipping school, receiving poor grades, staying out until "all hours of the morning," and coming home "stoned." Laura added that Keith was from her first marriage. His father had reportedly "disappeared" when Keith was four and had not been heard from since. She married Jim when Keith was five years old, and they had a second son, Davey, four years later. It was Jim's first marriage. After gathering a few more details during our phone call, we set up a family session for a week later.

Session 1: Do I Know What I'm Doing?

Laura, Jim, and Keith were present at the first session. We agreed that, given the reasons for therapy and that Davey was just six, it was not necessary for him to attend. I was aware that from a classic family-systems perspective, I was breaking a central rule that all family members should be present. Just one session in and I was already wondering, "Do I know what I'm doing?" and "What would Carl Whitaker (who advocated seeing entire families) say?"

Laura explained that Keith's behavior was taking a toll on the family. She worked as a nurse, which meant that her days were very busy. Most weekdays, while at work, Laura would get multiple calls from Keith's school. She would hear her named paged over the intercom system, cringe, and say to herself, "Not again!" The calls usually concerned the same issue. Keith would arrive at his school, where he was a sophomore, but wander the hallways instead of going to class. Sometimes he would make it to class, other times not. When he was in class, he did not do schoolwork, resulting in poor grades. Keith had an IEP (individualized education program) due to work incompletion that stipulated that he could not be suspended for missing class, leaving the school few other options. Jim explained that the stress on Laura had "pushed her past the breaking point." She was not sleeping well, was increasingly short-tempered, and was at risk of losing her job.

Jim worked for a telecommunications company. Because he had been in Keith's life since he was five, he struggled to understand how "an easy-going, loving boy" had come into so much trouble. Jim added that Keith's behavior had steadily deteriorated over the past three years to the point that they had sought help from a therapist 15 months earlier. I asked Jim what they had taken away from that experience of therapy. He replied, "It wasn't helpful. We were told that Keith had something called 'ODD' [oppositional defiant disorder], and his behavior would only get worse. The therapist also told us to put Keith in a home – some kind of place for delinquent kids – he was vague about it. The whole thing was confusing." Jim continued, "He also said that because I was Keith's stepfather and Laura was his biological parent, she should be the one to handle consequences." I asked Jim what parts of the therapist's advice he agreed with, if any. He replied, "I didn't agree with much of anything. But the guy was supposed to be an expert. We had another appointment scheduled, but when we got home Laura and I looked at each and said, 'No way are we going back.' So, we cancelled the appointment and that was it until we decided to try therapy again." I let all three family members know that I appreciated them coming to see me and that I would do my best to help them.

Keith was largely silent during the first session. He sat with his head down, hair over his eyes, and at times appeared asleep. I wondered if he was "high," but when I asked him a question he would raise his head long enough to answer it before retreating. His answers were brief but clear. He showed little outward emotion except for occasionally flashing a frown or furrowed eyebrow when he disagreed with something his mom or Jim said. Later in the session, I met with Keith individually in the hope that he might open up. But he remained steadfast in his demeanor, revealing little more than when his parents were present.

As the first session came to an end, I brought them all back together and asked what the family hoped would be different as a result of coming to see me. Laura answered first: "Keith will be 16 in two months and if this is the way it's going to be, then he won't be living with us. Not to sound insensitive, but I don't care where he goes at that point. It's not fair to me, Jim, or Davey. It hurts me to say this, but he'll be out of our home, and it will be up to him to make it on his own. I want him to get his act together, but if he doesn't he'll be out. I've had it." Jim agreed with Laura but was less specific: "Something has to change. We're worn out. I don't want him to be homeless, but we can't continue like this. He has to change."

I watched Keith's reactions to Laura and Jim's statements. He did not change his posture. He did not look up or interject. When I asked Keith what he hoped for, he fell silent. After a few moments, I asked if he agreed or disagreed with what he had heard. Keith only shrugged his shoulders. When I wondered aloud what Keith's nonverbal response meant, he did not flinch. A second family therapy appointment was set for eight days later.

Comment: The Situation is Serious, But Not Hopeless. I was nervous following the first session, unsure whether I could help the family. There were moments that I thought, "I don't know what to do." As I completed my session notes I realized that part of my anxiety was because I did not have a clear idea of what the family wanted. I had asked each of them, but when I received vague responses, I did not follow up. I needed to simplify and focus. I knew how to be directive in therapy because I had been well trained in that area, and yet my intuition told me that if we were going to get anywhere, it would have to be a collaborative process. The influence of the "third wave" therapies (O'Hanlon, 1999) that emphasized collaboration, strengths, and the like had found its way into my strategic thinking.

Session 2: Understanding the Pattern

In the second session, I asked more about Laura and Jim's concerns. They reiterated their worries about Keith's behavior at school, and also described another troublesome pattern. Keith would come home after school, then around 5:00 p.m. he would "disappear." He stayed out until 2:00 a.m. most nights. Laura and Jim would go to bed around 10:30 p.m. only to be awakened by sounds of

Keith creeping across the hardwood floors to his bedroom. On occasion, Laura would get up and attempt to speak with Keith, who frequently reeked of marijuana. Keith would roll over and go to sleep and try to ignore Laura's pleas to understand what was happening.

What Laura and Jim wanted most was for Keith to go to school regularly and, in Laura's words, "get an education to make something of his life." The preference was for him to attend college or get a job in a profession that could turn into a career. They also wanted Keith to at least tell them where he was going and be home by curfew. Lastly, they wanted him to "enjoy life without using pot." When I asked Keith what he would like to have change in his life or family, he remained silent.

Comment: I now felt clearer about their concerns and the purpose of therapy. The tension between Laura, Jim, and Keith was palpable. I was aware that Keith would be kicked out of his house in a matter of weeks unless things changed. I did my best to convey to Laura and Jim that I understood the gravity of their situation. I then asked, "How committed are you to doing whatever it takes to try and get things going in a better direction?" Each responded that they would do "whatever it takes" but, if things did not change, Keith would be on the streets in a few weeks. Keith remained quiet during the discussion. I wrapped up the session by asking the family to come back the following week. I restated their words, "*whatever it takes*," to solidify their commitment to getting things on track.

Session 3: Whatever It Takes

From a strategic family therapy perspective, most often it is the therapist who requests that the family make a commitment to do whatever is asked of them. The therapist will say some variation of, "You need to do this for your family." In this situation, however, it was the parents who stated they would do "whatever it takes." I felt I could balance directiveness with collaboration, the latter of which would largely come by offering the family opportunities to modify the forthcoming plan.

The third session began with revisiting and securing the couple's commitment to do "whatever it takes."

Bob: I've thought a lot about what is happening with your family. It's clear to me that you want what's best. I also think I'm clear about your concerns, Laura and Jim. And although you've kept mostly to yourself, Keith, I believe you want things to be different, and better. As I understand it, we're at a critical point now – things are close to falling apart. Continuing as is, is not a good plan. *(Looking at Laura and Jim)* Each of you has said you are willing to do *whatever it takes* to improve things. Keith, until proven otherwise, I'm going to assume that your silence means you agree with that idea. Before we talk about what we're going to do, I want to say one last thing. We're talking about your lives. No matter what we discuss and agree about right now, the biggest decision will be about what you actually do when you leave here today. I'm going to ask that each person do their part. I'll be specific. At the same time, if what we're talking about doesn't fit for you I ask that you speak up and offer an alternative so the old patterns that are not working aren't repeated. How does that sound?

(Laura and Jim stated their agreement. Keith remained silent)

Next, I began to offer a new frame, a different way of thinking about the current situation – one that, if effective, would make the most of the couple's commitment and concurrently perturb the system.

Bob: Laura, you have stated that if Keith does not change his behavior very soon, he will be out of the house. Is that still how you feel? *(Laura nodded in the affirmative.)* Jim, do you agree with Laura? *(Jim agreed.)* Keith, this would be a great opportunity to hear about how you see things. What would you like to share about the situation we've been talking about? *(Keith shrugged his shoulders.)* Okay, if at any time you would like to chime in, please do. Let's get to work. You all know that here at YIN [Youth in Need] we work with many homeless teens. One of the things I've learned from these youth is that a different kind of education from what is learned in school is necessary when it comes to survival. *(Looking at Keith)* I understand that you've missed quite a bit of school this year but, as it stands, there are things you're going to need to learn to make it on your own. The basics like how to cook, some first aid, how to keep yourself safe – things like that. Our mission, then, is to prepare you to take care of yourself. *(Looking at Laura and Jim)* Does that make sense? *(Laura and Jim nodded in agreement – they still seemed ready to do "whatever it takes.")* Okay, let's talk about the best way for you, Keith, to get the education you need to live on your own, on the streets.

Comment: If change was going to occur with the already existing patterns that surrounded and maintained the problem, the new frame had to be one that the parents could agree on. Of the many threads that could have been pursued, I decided to remain with the strategy the couple had presented, namely, that Keith would not live at home past age 16 without changes to his behavior. My hope was to redirect their energy away from evicting Keith from the house and toward the new idea of educating him to live on the streets and take care of himself. With agreement around the new frame, I felt their follow-through with the forthcoming plan would be further enhanced.

At that point, the following interchange took place. I continued to observe Keith, who maintained a fixed gaze on the floor, until the last part of the conversation.

Bob: One of the first things you mentioned, Laura, was how often you were being called at work about Keith missing class. Am I getting that right?

Laura: Right, I get called several times a day.

Bob: Okay. And Jim, do I have it right that the previous therapist advised that Laura handle consequences at home?

Jim: Yeah, he said the biological parent should be the one handling consequences for Keith.

Bob: It seems to me that that idea hasn't worked too well.

Jim: It hasn't.

Laura: Not one bit.

Bob: Right. You're in this together. You are both parents to Keith. Jim, you've been a parent to Keith since he was five years old. You've cared for him through the good times and the bad.

Jim: I feel like I have and maybe I can do more.

Bob: I agree and appreciate your commitment to your family. Laura, are you ready to have Jim do more?

Laura: Without a doubt… do you have something in mind?

Bob: I do. Let's start with school. Jim, how available are you during the day should there be a need to contact you?

Jim: Very. I'm very available. My job is flexible with just a couple of exceptions. I have two standing meetings a week but can be reached easily. Laura's never had trouble getting ahold of me.

Bob: Wonderful. It's time for Jim to be the contact person for school so we can relieve some of the pressure on you *(Looking at Laura.)* Okay? *(Laura nodded her head in agreement.)* Jim, are you for that?

Jim: Of course. I'm happy to do whatever is necessary.

Bob: All right. *(To Laura)* Can you please call the school tomorrow and make sure they know that Jim is the person to contact going forward?

Laura: Yes. That's easy to do.

Bob: Great. There's one more thing. When you call the school, tell whomever you talk with that unless there is some fear about his safety, they should call just once per day. That call should come at the end of the day with one piece of information – the number of minutes Keith missed from each class for the entire day. So, even though Keith has missed parts of three classes – 10 minutes from one, 20 for another, and 25 from a third – there would be a total of 55 minutes missed. Or, if it's easier for the school, they can just give you one total number for the entire day. Neither the school nor you need to be exact – just approximate the time missed. Does that make sense?

Laura: Yes. I get it.

Jim: Yep.

Bob: All right, now let's remember that if Keith is not in class, he's not learning. He needs to learn about how to take care of himself – we have to make sure he gets that information. So, Keith may have a health course, but he's not there regularly and he's missing vital information. When we work with youth who are homeless here at YIN, we teach life skills. That's what Keith needs. Are we ready to move on?

(Laura and Jim nodded in agreement. Keith continued to look sullen.)

Bob: I understand that Keith takes off most nights before dinner and doesn't return until very late, sometimes the next morning. But you know when he gets home. And that will be the time he gets the education he needs. When Keith gets home, no matter the time, the both of you will get up, go to Keith's room, and study with him for the amount of time that he missed in school that day. It will be hard on the two of you at first, but you will adjust to it. When you're exhausted and have to get up for work in just a few hours, you'll have to remember that Keith needs to be educated about living on the streets and fending for himself.

Jim: We can do that, but how do we study with him? He never brings books home.

Bob: That's a great question. We have to keep in mind that the kind of education Keith needs to survive can't be found in his textbooks. This is where your life experience and education will benefit Keith. Let's start with Laura. Do you have some nursing books around? Maybe something with basic first-aid or self-care information in it?

Laura: Tons of stuff. I still have books from my program 20 years ago.

Bob: Fantastic. Take a look at what you have when you get home and pick out a couple things that you think might be helpful to Keith. *(To Jim)* What could you share with Keith? Think in terms of practical knowledge that you might have learned before leaving home.

Jim: I was just thinking… We have a Time-Life series of books on camping, survival skills, and if I remember, basics of cooking. It's like a book-of-the-month club.

Bob: That is just the kind of education he needs.

Comment: As the discussion progressed, I could see Keith's face turning red. I did not know what it meant until he lifted his head and looked toward his mother. It was then that I could see his face was flush with anger. This was the most emotional expression I had seen from him. He did not say a word, but something he had heard was producing a "You Said *What*?" moment! When I invited Keith to share his thoughts, he returned his gaze to the floor. The conversation continued.

Laura: We've tried to talk to him when he's come in late and sometimes he's high and it seems pointless. Or he just rolls over and ignores us and goes to sleep.

Bob: You've done a great job of trying to get through to Keith, and he's now going to need you more than ever. Because learning takes commitment. Even if he tries to go to sleep it's going to take him a few minutes. And with both of you talking and sharing information that will be challenging to sleep through. But there's something else. There's some research that suggests that we may even learn things while we sleep. So, don't worry if he falls asleep. Just finish out the time as planned. *(Looking at Keith)* Who knows what you might learn without even trying?

Laura and Jim seemed satisfied with the idea. Keith expressed his displeasure by picking at a cushion on the couch and letting out a deep sigh.

Collaboration to Increase Follow-Through. It was at this point that I invited feedback about the plan. I was not renegotiating the focus of therapy, only how Keith could receive the education he needs.

Bob: Let's pause for a moment to check in about what we've discussed so far. Because what I'm asking is a departure from what you've been doing, if there's anything about our plan that you are uncomfortable with or want to tweak, now's the time.

Laura: To be perfectly honest, I'm not thrilled about getting up at 2:00 in the morning or whatever because I have to be at work at 6:00 a.m. But if it's going to get him to take care of himself, then I'll do it.

Jim: I always wake up when Keith comes home because of the squeaky floors. And I usually don't get right back to sleep, so it's no problem for me. I'll sleep better knowing that we did something to help him.

Bob: It sounds like we're in-sync. Keith, there's still time for your input. What would you like to add into the plan?

Keith lifted his head and looked at me. His face was still red with what I interpreted as a continuation of his anger, although it also could have indicated frustration. To my question he replied, "Nothing."

Practicing the Plan. The final part of the third session was used to practice what we had discussed. I wanted to be sure that Laura and Jim were clear about what I was asking them to do. I brought in a dictionary to serve as "educational material." I then set up a scenario and asked the couple to practice with me.

Bob: Since it's now 8:45 at night, let's move forward to tomorrow and go through the plan. Laura, you will make arrangements with the school for Jim to be the one called about Keith missing class. And the school will know to only call once, near the end of the day, with a total number of minutes Keith missed class for the day.

Laura: Right.

Bob: Let's assume it's tomorrow evening, the school called with a report, and Keith missed only a few minutes of his classes – only seven minutes for the entire day. Now, Keith has been out most of the night and he gets back home at 1:30 in the morning. *(Looking at Laura and Jim)* The two of you get up and grab some reading material you've set aside. You then go to Keith's room, or wherever he is, and you begin to read aloud to him for seven minutes.

Laura: Got it.

Jim: Me, too.

Bob: I have a dictionary we can use to practice. Let's start at the top with the very first entry, which is the letter "A." Laura, let's have you begin, then Jim will do the next entry, which is the word "aardvark." I'll keep track of time.

Laura read through the many uses of the letter "A." The three of us laughed at some of its uses and there was an occasional "I didn't know that" from one of us. During this time, I continued to observe Keith's reactions. He stirred, shifted in his seat, and sighed. Several times I said some variation of "It's nice to know that we can learn," "There is much so much to learn," "I wonder what is being learned now," and "How much more will be learned when the readings come from books on safety and first aid?" These statements were Ericksonian suggestions, not necessarily about first-aid or the alphabet – the ideas that we can learn, that there is much to learn, and how much more will be learned?

It was a Tuesday evening and we scheduled the next session for nine days later to allow time for the process we had outlined. I felt comfortable that Keith would return home and be confronted with the ordeal we had constructed as opposed to pushing back and staying out even longer.

Comment: The Use of an Ordeal. Milton Erickson (1965; also see Haley, 1973, 1984; and Chapter 11, this volume) often prescribed ordeals – tasks or situations – that his patients despised and found equal to or more distressing than the problems they experienced. The aim was to link the task's difficulty to the problem behavior and, in turn, make continuing the behavior difficult. When successful, the ordeals would lead his patients to engage in the behaviors or symptoms that they had struggled with (e.g., sleeping, reducing alcohol consumption, etc.). They would arrive at the conclusion that giving up the problem was a better choice than maintaining it and facing an ordeal.

In this case, I predicted that the prospect of having to study with his parents would be more agonizing for Keith than attending his classes. It would also be an ordeal for the parents to deal with him at 2 a.m. My hope was, of course, that the ordeal would never be played out. However, if it did, the pattern around the problem would be disrupted by the changes to its sequence. I also knew that sometimes families do not do agreed-upon tasks, which can also reveal further information. So whether they did the task or did not, whether it failed or was a partial success, I was of the belief that no matter what happened when the family left my office, something more would be learned about the problem.

Session 4: Strangely Nice

The family arrived on time for their 6:00 p.m. appointment the following Tuesday. As soon as he sat down, Keith began to look at the floor. Whereas Laura and Jim appeared to be in good spirits, as evidenced by their laughing about something that happened on the drive to the session, there was no indication of how things were with Keith.

Bob: How has the last week or so been, including six days of school for Keith?

Laura: (First looking at Jim, then to me) Well, I called the school last Wednesday. That didn't take long. Initially they were confused, but when I explained what I wanted in more detail they agreed.

Bob: Okay. And they agreed to call Jim, just once per school day, with the number of minutes Keith missed for that day?

Laura: They did.

Jim: But here's the thing: I haven't been called once. Not one time.

Bob: And they had your number right…

Jim: …Yeah, they literally did NOT call. I actually called the school last Friday to double-check. He hadn't missed one minute.

Bob: Now I'm confused. The school knew what to do, but they didn't need to call? He has not missed one minute of school?

My remarks were apparently enough to prompt a response from Keith. He was quick to clarify that what was reported was true.

Keith: I didn't miss any school.

Bob: (Looking at Keith) That's impressive. I'm actually a little stunned. I thought the amount of time you missed each day might vary – but going straight to zero, wow. How did you do that?

Keith shrugged his shoulders and offered no further clarification.

Bob: It's okay if you don't have anything further to say. Sometimes I don't feel like talking either. Thank you for clarifying for me what happened. Maybe something will come to you later that you'd like to say out loud. If not, that's okay, too. We can still appreciate the effort you've made. *(Looking to Laura and Jim)* What do you think is going on here?

Laura: I have no idea. And before I forget, he was also home for a few nights when he usually would have been out running around.

Bob: Home like around dinnertime or later in the evening?

Laura: Both. We all watched a movie together the other night, which hasn't happened in over a year. It was nice. And Keith played a board game with Davey. I can't remember the last time that happened.

Jim: It's been strangely nice, if that makes any sense. Every day I'm waiting for the call. Thinking, today is the day. At first, I thought they had to have my number wrong and that Laura would call and say, "The school is still calling me!" But that wasn't the case.

Laura: (Laughing) Yeah, I called Jim the first three days and said, "Why haven't you updated me?" He said, "No one has called." So, I was wondering where the breakdown was.

Bob: What I'm hearing is that there have been other good things happening outside of Keith attending school. What difference has that made in the family?

Laura: The stress level has gone way down.

Jim: A lot.

Bob: How so?

Laura: We're talking to each other instead of yelling. It's, dare I say, peaceful.

Bob: You're all talking with each other more…

Jim: …We're talking and just enjoying being around each other.

Bob: That does sound peaceful. And one way that you can tell the stress has gone down is by you all talking with each other?

Laura: Right.

Bob: Keith, anything you'd like to add?

Keith: I don't know. I guess.

Bob: About?

Keith: There's no yelling.

Bob: Okay. I appreciate the feedback from each of you. So, on one hand there's much to feel good about and also maybe some reason to proceed with caution.

Laura: Exactly, I'm cautiously happy.

Bob: That's a good way to put it.

Laura: Yeah, I'm thrilled about how things have been but still worried.

Bob: Makes sense to me.

Jim: I feel the same way. I wish I knew why he's done so much better.

Bob: I mentioned that here at YIN we see many youth Keith's age. But it's not that often we see such a dramatic change from one week to the next. That has me wondering if Keith is growing into the 16-year-old he will soon be, chronologically. Maybe he's maturing, thinking of the impact of what he does on others, just being more thoughtful. That's the kind of thing that some teenagers don't start thinking about until they are young adults. It's possible that Keith is already becoming more of a responsible young man and realizing that things can be very different going forward for him, and for all of you. Maybe he's beginning to leave the old behavior behind.

Laura: We don't know. But being able to talk about things is huge and as far as we can tell he hasn't been getting high.

Bob: Maybe it's another example that Keith may be looking at things differently. As it stands, the sample size is small right now. So, is it possible this is just a phase? Possibly. Maintaining the plan is important. Keith will be 16 soon and we've discussed what that could mean...

Laura: We've talked about that.

Bob: There's no reason to doubt Keith that he is growing into a more thoughtful young man. But, there's also no room to be naïve here. I'm hearing that both of you are still willing and ready to do whatever it takes to prepare Keith for the next phase of his life. If trouble returns with school, you know what to do. If Keith maintains his new course, you can help him to explore his future and dreams.

Jim: I look forward to that.

Bob: To talking with Keith about his future?

Jim: Absolutely. He's got a real aptitude for creating things with his hands. I'd love to help him look at some career choices. Those are enjoyable talks compared to the ones we've been having for the last couple of years.

Bob: It's exciting to me whenever I hear people talk about pursuing their hopes and dreams.

Comment: Optimism and Caution. Because Laura and Jim needed to know they had done everything they could before having Keith leave the home, I was confident that they would carry out the task. What I did not expect was that Keith would attend every minute of school. With the positive change in school came additional "ripples" including Keith being around the home more, the family spending time together, and talking to each other. There was a growing sense of optimism.

There was also reason to be cautious about the change. If Keith were to revert to his previous behavior he would be on his own in a few weeks. I commented that the "sample size" was small and speculated that Keith's change may just be a phase. Strategic therapists often anticipate and even prescribe relapses (setbacks) (Weakland, Fisch, Watzlawick, & Bodin, 1974). I used a variation of this idea by acknowledging Keith's forward movement and simultaneously suggesting it could be just a phase and it was not the time to be naïve. My hope in mentioning a possible relapse was that the new behavior would be sustained.

From Boredom to a Future. The remainder of the session focused on indications that the improvement with Keith was more than happenstance. Laura and Jim stated that if Keith were to continue to attend classes for two more weeks they would consider the change "real" and that Keith was "serious" about his future. A comment by Laura, near the end of the session, piqued my curiosity about the advancement of hope with the situation.

Laura: Keith told me the other night that he's bored in school. He said he wants to learn but that the teachers keep going over the same things. My first thought was, huh? I mean, he was a good student until about three years ago, then his grades took a dive. That's when we got him an IEP, thinking that he just needed more support getting work done. Is boredom really part of all this?

Bob: (Looking at Laura) That's interesting. Keith's the only one who can answer if boredom is part of the equation. He wouldn't be the first high-school student to not feel connected to his studies.

Laura: Well, that's true!

Keith looked up at his mom as she spoke, and continued to do so even as I responded. His face was no longer flush. In fact, there appeared to be a hint of affection toward her. I was a little tepid about engaging Keith since my previous attempts had not gone well. So, I decided to look at the floor, as he had done many times, before I continued with my comment.

Bob: I'm wondering out loud here. Sometimes the reasons we do things are because we just haven't yet figured out a better way. It's only when we shake things up a little that we are able to see things differently. I think it was a brave thing for Keith to tell you he was bored, and we should accept it at face value. And whether it's now, tonight, or in a few days, I'm hopeful that he will say more about how about how those who love and care about him can help him.

After I was done, I continued to look down, careful not to add to the pressure of the moment. Fortunately, Keith was ready to engage.

Keith: I can pass the GED [General Education Diploma – a high-school equiv-alency exam]. I want to study art and can't do that at school. Plus, there are too many cliques.

Laura: GED? I'm not sure you even qualify...

Keith: I will in a few weeks when I'm 16. You guys say you want me to think about the future. Well, I am.

I was hopeful about the conversation that was taking place, and let it play out as long as possible. However, we had run out of time and I had another client waiting. I asked Keith if he would be willing to share more details of his idea with his mom and Jim that night. I also asked that the parents provide Keith with the opportunity to fully explain what he was thinking before pro-viding their point of view. Everyone agreed to my request. I then asked what time the conversation would occur. They settled on 9:00 p.m., after Davey was in bed. A fifth session was scheduled for eight days later.

Session 5: Tears of Joy

From the start of the fifth session it was evident that further changes had occurred. To begin, Keith sat forward in his seat, made eye contact, and seemed eager to get the conversation started.

Laura: We're still on track. No problems whatsoever with school. Keith has been to every minute of every class.

Jim: It's that, plus he's just like a different person. He's talking with us more.

Bob: That does sound different and wonderful. Just one more question before we talk about the plan. Keith, what can you tell me about how things changed? I'm learning here as well, and I want to understand as best as I can what's happened.

Keith: One thing is they stopped pressuring me about school. I'm almost 16, but they were acting like I was 12. They're listening to me.

Bob: And that is different than before?

Keith: Totally.

Bob: Do you feel like this is a change for the good?

Keith: Huh-huh (*said affirmatively, looking toward Laura*).

Laura: (*Visibly tearful*) These are tears of joy. I can't believe where we are now compared to a few weeks ago.

They went on to report that after the last session, they had gone home and talked. Keith had agreed to study, finish the school year, and prepare for and take the GED test.

Jim: I feel like a weight has been lifted off the whole family. We are talking every night. And Keith asked us to help him study!

Laura: We are in a very good place now.

The four of us agreed that we would take a break from therapy for the summer and reevaluate things in August. I let them know that if something came up sooner they could call and schedule an appointment.

Follow-Up

In early August Laura called me. She expressed excitement that Keith had passed his GED. He had enrolled in community college for the fall and agreed to take two general education courses in addition to art. Keith had begun working at a local electronics store in June and the family had purchased another car, so he would have transportation to work and school. We jointly decided that a further family therapy session was not needed at the time. I invited Laura to schedule a session if in the future there were any challenges.

Just before the call ended, she made an interesting comment: "I remember you talking about Keith needing a different education to survive on the streets. You know, I think Jim and I are the ones who got an education. We learned how to handle a situation that was unexpected and new to us. It makes sense when you think about it. I mean, I have to get continuing education as a nurse. Parents need it, too. We never stop learning."

Reflections

As I have gained more experience, I have become more comfortable responding to whatever emerges from interactions with clients. I continue to employ structure, but in a different way. I work with clients to determine goals, explore their ideas about change, and about potential pathways for achieving the results they want. I also measure the "fit" of the approach I am using and the "effect" or benefit of services (Bertolino, 2014, 2017; Rousmaniere, 2017). We will make errors and through reflection we can develop plans to improve.

References

Bertolino, B. (1999). *Therapy with troubled teenagers: Rewriting young lives in progress.* New York: Wiley.

Bertolino, B. (2014). *Thriving on the front lines: A guide to strengths-based youth care work.* New York: Routledge.

Bertolino, B. (2017). *Effective counseling and psychotherapy: An evidence-based approach.* New York: Springer.

Erickson, M.H. (1965). The use of symptoms as an integral part of psychotherapy. *American Journal of Clinical Hypnosis, 8,* 57–65.

Haley. J. (1973). *Uncommon therapy: The psychiatric techniques of Milton H. Erickson, M.D.* New York: Norton.

Haley, J. (1984). *Ordeal therapy: Unusual ways to change behavior.* San Francisco: Jossey-Bass.

Haley, J. (1987). *Problem-solving therapy* (2nd ed.). San Francisco: Jossey-Bass.

Hoyt, M.F. (Ed.). (1994). *Constructive therapies.* New York: Guilford Press.

Hoyt, M.F. (Ed.). (1996). *Constructive therapies 2.* New York: Guilford Press.

Madanes, C. (1981). *Strategic family therapy.* San Francisco: Jossey-Bass.

O'Hanlon, W.H. (1987). *Taproots: Underlying principles of Milton H. Erikson's therapy and hypnosis.* New York: Norton.

O'Hanlon, B. (1999). What's the story? Narrative therapy and the third wave of psychotherapy. In O'Hanlon, S., & Bertolino, B. (Eds.). *Evolving possibilities: Selected papers of Bill O'Hanlon* (pp. 205–220). Philadelphia, PA: Brunner/Mazel. [paperback edition, New York: Routledge, 2014]

O'Hanlon, W.H., & Hexum A.L. (1990). *An uncommon casebook: The complete clinical work of Milton H. Erickson, M.D.* New York: Norton.

O'Hanlon, W.H., & Weiner-Davis, M. (2003). *In search of solutions: A new direction in psychotherapy* (2nd ed.). New York: Norton.

Rousmaniere, T. (2017). *Deliberate practice for psychotherapists: A guide to improving clinical effectiveness.* New York: Routledge.

Watzlawick, P., Weakland, J.H., & Fisch, R. (1974). *Change: Principles of problem formation and problem resolution.* New York: Norton.

Weakland, J.H., Fisch, R., Watzlawick, P., & Bodin, A. (1974). Brief therapy: Focused problem resolution. *Family Process, 13*(2), 141–167.

CHAPTER 4

On a Small Island off the Coast of Texas

Monte Bobele

In this chapter, I will present five examples of *You Said What?* moments. Two are examples of my own work, and three are from my mentors at the Galveston Family Institute (GFI), which has since moved to Houston and been renamed the Houston Galveston Institute (HGI). All of the examples are from work done on Galveston Island. HGI is one of three surviving original family therapy institutes, along with the Ackerman Family Institute and the Mental Research Institute.

The Galveston Family Institute

In the spring of 1977, I was sitting in my private practice office in Houston when a yellow flyer arrived announcing an upcoming workshop in Galveston. The reason that GFI workshop attracted me was that it said that it would "be of particular interest to therapists acquainted with the clinical work of Milton Erickson, Jay Haley, the Milan group, the Palo Alto group, and Carl Whitaker." As it happened, I had been introduced to Jay Haley by Jerry Osborne, the director of the University of Houston Counseling Center, when I was an intern a few years earlier. Jerry stopped by my office one day and dropped a book on my desk saying, "I think you'll find some interesting stuff in here that you will like." Thus, was I introduced to Haley by way of *The Power Tactics of Jesus Christ* (Haley, 1969a).

Haley led me to Milton Erickson and an interest in hypnosis (Haley, 1971, 1973). Shortly after I had begun private practice, another friend handed me the Milan group's just-published *Paradox and Counterparadox* (Palazzoli et al., 1978). In fact, I was in my office reading the Milan team's book when the invitation to the GFI workshop arrived. The names of the workshop presenters were unknown to me at the time: Harry Goolishian, George Pulliam, Paul Dell, and Harlene Kivell (later she reclaimed her maiden name: Anderson). I was intrigued. I didn't think anyone in my vicinity was doing work based on these ideas. I got on the phone, called the Flagship Hotel and immediately booked a room for the duration of the workshop.

That weekend, I was fascinated by the lectures and the videos that were presented by the faculty of the newly founded GFI. All of them at the time were also on the faculty of the University of Texas Medical Branch (UTMB) in Galveston – Texas' oldest medical school, founded in 1892. I later learned that UTMB was one of the first family therapy treatment, training, and research facilities in the country.[1] Harlene has recently recalled the innovative work that was going on there by the time she arrived in the early '70s (Duvall et al., 2015; Duvall et al., 2016). As Harlene said in these interviews, "Harry and his colleagues … had been involved in family therapy research and training since the late 1950s" (Duvall et al., 2016, p. 61).

Many of the examples of *You Said What?* moments in this book are the result of the creative work of the early family therapy theorists such as the Palo Alto group, more commonly known as the Mental Research Institute (MRI). It was at that workshop where I saw several videos that intrigued me. My first taste of these new ways of working was at GFI's first public workshop in March 1978. In fact, most of the two-day workshop was a revelatory *You Said What?* experience for me.

In one of the videos, Paul Dell was working with a young woman who was referred to him for help with her poorly controlled diabetes. As you will see from my first example, Paul's joining with her around her unwillingness to be pushed around by her illness rather than collaborating with traditional approaches of psychoeducation was uncommon for the times. Well, I was hooked. I did not understand all that was presented over that workshop weekend, but I wanted to.

At the closing cocktail party at Harry Goolishian's house (a GFI tradition), I cornered Harry and Harlene and asked what I could do to learn more about this new way of looking at therapy. They invited me to the coming year's weekly externship program. So, the following year, I commuted every Thursday to Galveston for a day-long training in family therapy with Harry and his crew. At the end of that year, over drinks, I told Harry that I thought I was beginning to get it, but I thought I needed something else. Harry said, with that twinkle in his eye, "Well, it's kind of like psychoanalysis. If once a week is not enough, then maybe you need daily treatment." He invited me to apply for a full-time postdoctoral fellowship. So, the following year, I closed my practice, moved to Galveston Island, and became immersed in a new way of thinking about problems, clients, and therapy.

My year as a post-doctoral fellow at GFI opened my eyes to many ways of thinking about and doing therapy. I was fortunate to be able to work with Harry, Harlene, George Pulliam, and Paul Dell during that year. Paul was Harry's protégé and supervised a number of cases I worked on. During that second year, I had many interesting, unusual, challenging cases.

My Own Early *You Said What?* Cases

The first was the case of a woman who had arrived at GFI afraid to go home, and afraid to not go home, to an abusive partner. The second involved a young teenager who was threatening to murder a woman she thought was responsible for the death of her premature baby. They were originally described in a paper published in the *Journal of Marital and Family Therapy* (Bobele, 1987). The paper presented a rationale for unusual, somewhat perilous interventions based on the work of John Weakland (Weakland et al., 1974) and his colleagues at MRI. I must admit that for several months after the publication of the paper, I was worried that I might face angry critiques from feminists and "experts" in the fields of family violence and couples' therapy. At the time, I was on the faculty at Texas Tech University in a department that was populated by a number of women who identified as feminists and were frequently at odds with the family therapy faculty, most of whom were men. Context is everything.

I was quite surprised when a letter arrived from Al Gurman, the editor of *JMFT*, including a paper that he planned to publish that was highly critical of my work. The authors were a lawyer/psychologist and a social worker who took issue with the ethical/legal problems they thought were evident in my paper (Woody & Woody, 1988). They all but called for my license to be revoked. Gurman invited me to respond to their critique in whatever way I wanted. He assured me that he would publish whatever I submitted. At the time, I was working on an article on a systemic approach to the treatment of hiccups (Bobele, 1989). I thought briefly about submitting that hiccups paper to *JMFT* because it applied the same principles to a much more prosaic problem and would not prompt the type of critique the Woodys had made. The point, I thought, was that if I demonstrated the use of similar approaches in a less controversial case, the same interventions (symptom prescription, reframing, etc.) would surely be seen in a less controversial light. Doing so, I thought, might have been too subtle a rejoinder. In the end, I sought the advice of colleagues (Insoo Kim Berg, Richard Fisch, Harry Goolishian, Brad Keeney, and John Weakland) and decided to write a more direct response (Bobele, 1988). That series of articles, critiques, and letters to the editor have become part of ethics courses at several universities since (Bobele, 1987, 1988; Woody & Woody, 1988; Weakland, 1988; Woody, 1990.). I will return to this critique later, in the Editors' Conclusion chapter, because the issues raised are relevant for several of the cases presented in this volume. The two *You Said What?* examples from the *JMFT* article appear later in this chapter.

Illustrations of *You Said What?*

These stories follow from Bateson's (1972; Ruesch & Bateson, 1951) ideas that were elaborated by the original MRI team that all behavior and meaning construction is interactional. Most elegantly articulated in their seminal paper on focused problem resolution, Weakland, Fisch, Watzlawick, and Bodin (1974) described a problematic interactional cycle where participants reciprocally escalated ineffective efforts to change one another's behavior in an attempt to solve their mutual problem. What was revolutionary for the field of psychotherapy was their bypassing any need for etiologic psychological explanations for problems beyond the understanding of the positive feedback loop that maintained the problematic situation. Their recommended solution was deceptively simple – *interrupt the problematic cycle*:

> We see the resolution of problems as primarily requiring a substitution of behavior patterns so as to interrupt the vicious, positive feedback circles. Other less destructive and less distressing behaviors are potentially open to the patient and involved family members at all times. It is usually impossible, however, for them to change from their rigidly patterned, traditional, unsuccessful problem-solving behavior to more appropriate behavior on their own initiative. This is especially likely when such usual behavior is culturally supported, as is often the case: Everyone *knows* that people should do their best to encourage and cheer up a loved one who is sad and depressed. Such behavior is both "right" and "logical" – but often it just doesn't work.
>
> (Weakland et al., 1974, pp. 149–150)

The following case vignettes exemplify how the therapists' interventions were aimed at finding ways, albeit unusual ways, to help people interrupt positive feedback loops by substituting other behavioral patterns. In each case, you will likely observe that the intervention, the *You Said What?* moment, follows the observation of Weakland et al. (1974) that what seemed to be the "right" thing to do, the most "logical," was often precisely what therapists needed to avoid.

Example 1: "I Don't Want to Be a Fool"

Paul Dell,[2] during his psychology internship at UTMB Galveston, was referred a "resistant" 18-year-old girl who had diabetes that had resulted in recurrent hospitalizations because she failed to maintain her diet. Her doctors requested the consultation to determine how this young woman could be motivated to follow her restrictive, but necessary, treatment plan. The woman, let's call her Deborah, described all of the troubles that she had with keeping her diabetes in control. Deborah related how all of the healthcare professionals involved with her had given her dire warnings about the consequences of not eating well, not exercising, not taking her medicine, and so on. While watching the video for the first time, I was struck, as was Paul (it turned out), how throughout her recounting of her care team's efforts to get her on the right track in managing her illness, Deborah maintained a proud grin on her face as if to say, "I defeated (frustrated, outlasted) all of them."

Finally, Paul said to her, "I could surely give you some good advice about how you should be taking care of yourself, but I don't want to be a fool. I could point out to you how continuing to do what you are doing will end up with your losing your legs, and fingers, and dying a premature death. But, I know I would be a fool to do that, and I don't want to be a fool." I noted that as Paul said this, seriously and with no trace of irony in his voice, Paul did have an ironic grin on his face that mirrored the grin Deborah had displayed since the interview begun.

As she began to protest and tell him that she had to do something about her dilemma, Paul continued to tell her, in effect, "I don't want to be a fool. I could give you some good advice and make excellent suggestions. But, all of the other doctors have done that, and you made fools out of them. I don't want to be a fool." Paul's smile continued to mirror her grin. As the session continued, Paul avoided being drawn into an advice-giving, life-saving position. He continued to talk with Deborah about how he knew that she knew what needed to be done, but that she was "too stubborn" (she agreed with that characterization) to let her life be controlled by her diabetes. By the end of the session, a strong therapeutic alliance had been established. Deborah moved from her position of "don't nothin' bother me" to one of agreeing that she would like to find a way to become more in charge of her life. A subsequent appointment was scheduled, and she eventually began to manage her diabetes in a healthier fashion.

Example 2: The Corrected Suicide Note

Through the late 1980s, the influences of the MRI and Milan therapists shook up the field of psychotherapy with their unusual, provocative, and unconventional approaches to working with difficult cases and in difficult circumstances. This was especially true at GFI.

I remember once when the client of one of my colleagues, Rob Horowitz[3] (one of the senior post-docs), showed up at GFI with a suicide note. The receptionist took the note to Rob, who was working in his office. Rob, a former high school English teacher in the South Bronx, carefully reviewed the note, made a number of marks and comments in red pencil on it, and scrawled a large C- at the top of the first page. Rob carried the graded suicide letter back out to the empty waiting room and sat down next to the client.

> I've read your suicide note and it shows a lot of promise. Unfortunately, the people who you want to read it are likely to be distracted by the poor grammar and punctuation errors in it. Your girlfriend, that you wrote this to, will not be able to appreciate the depth of your despair because your note is poorly written. It has misspellings, run-on sentences, and so on.

The best grade I can give you for this is a C-. I'll be happy to read your next draft. When you are finished with it, give it to the receptionist and she will bring it back for me to review.

I had been observing this interchange and was shocked and bemused at the same time. As Paul Watzlawick (1983) later quipped, therapy is too important to be taken seriously. I appreciated how earnestly Rob was taking this man's situation. Rob understood that the suicide note was a way of expressing his disappointments and despair. Rob took that so seriously that he wanted to help the client craft a credible note, one that was not marred by spelling, grammar, and usage errors. All the while, Rob had an enigmatic twinkle in his eye.

This process – write, review, critique – went on for a couple of hours. With each submission, the quality of the suicide note improved. Finally, Rob returned to the waiting room with the marked-up draft of the suicide note. Handing it to the young man, Rob said, again with the twinkling eye, "You have earned a B+ on this version of your work. This is a suicide note you can be proud of! Everyone who reads it will feel sorry for you and miss you. Your girlfriend will be especially sad that she mistreated you and will wish she had had an opportunity to make amends."

The client looked at Rob and said, "Thanks, I guess. You know, the last couple of hours, sitting here, writing and re-writing has forced me to evaluate why I was thinking about killing myself and what I was hoping it would accomplish. I've changed my mind about that, for now. I am going to have a conversation with my girlfriend about the things that I figured out while working on this note. I'll keep the note because it will remind me about how it is better to think carefully about suicide."

With a smile, and a twinkle in *his* eye, the client added, "And, boy, if I ever want to kill myself again, I'm not coming back here. You guys make it too hard!" The young man returned for his regularly scheduled visit the next week. Rob had given his client an unusual, but effective, way to express himself and perhaps to find some new understandings of himself.

Example 3: Stand By Your Man[4]

This case was seen during one of the weekly training groups at GFI. There were several post-masters' students, graduate practicum students, and four of the Institute's post-graduate fellows on the team.[5] The influences of the Milan team (Palazzoli et al., 1978) and the Mental Research Institute (Watzlawick, Weakland, and Fisch, 1974; Weakland et al., 1974) were prominent at that time. A local women's crisis shelter referred Sharon for counseling. The group decided that one of the other trainees and I would see her as co-therapists while the rest of the team observed from behind a one-way mirror.

She told us that Jerry, her live-in boyfriend of several years, had been an exceptionally kind and loving man, most of the time. He had been an excellent stepfather and her children cared for him as well. However, she described a long and difficult history of violent episodes with him. Her depiction of the cyclical nature of the relationship was that Jerry would become inexplicably insecure, followed by verbal assaults and then physical violence. After the situation calmed down, he became a doting, loving companion. She became very attuned to him and tried frequently to reassure him that he was her one and only. Nothing she tried worked to reassure Jerry and prevent the cycle from getting started. She had tried consulting with friends, family, clergymen, and the local crisis hotline; friends offered her a place to stay, battered women's shelter counselors had not been helpful to her, and so on. None of these help-givers provided her with the solution that would both stop the violence and continue the relationship.

In fact, these outside consultations that Sharon had only served to exacerbate Jerry's insecurities because he viewed these contacts as acts of disloyalty. The night before she was seen at GFI, her and Jerry's situation had arrived at a point where he had pulled a pistol out and fired two shots that landed near her. She did not think he intended to shoot her, but simply wanted to frighten her. Apparently, things cooled down after that for a while. Earlier in the day she had gone to work but remained worried about the explosiveness of the environment at home because the fights were becoming more violent.

My co-therapist and I were overwhelmed with this client's story and the challenges it presented. Any of the obvious steps we could have taken would have been more of what had already been tried and didn't work. After about 45 minutes, we told Sharon that we were going to take a break to consult with our team, "to put our heads together to figure out how to proceed." The entire team was energized to find a solution to the dilemma we had been presented with. Many different ideas were tossed around over an almost hour-long break. We recognized pieces of the paradoxical situation Sharon, Jerry, and their helpers were stuck in. The Milan team's formulation of tough cases proceeded from a thesis that systems were caught in a paradox, and their resolution was the prescription of an equally powerful counter-paradox. The typical Milan-style session (see Palazzoli et al., 1978) would result in the therapist returning to the client with a message that the team had composed behind the mirror and the therapist reading it to the client.

Following the lengthy team consultation behind the mirror, my co-therapist and I returned to the room with the resulting Milan-style prescriptive intervention:[6]

> We have been impressed with the enormity of the situation that you have been dealing with over the last few years. It is obvious to us that you love your boyfriend more than most women would be capable. In fact, most women would have, by now, given up on ever being able to convince such a man of the depth of their love and the amount of caring that exists. God knows that you have tried everything you know to do. In fact, you have

continually sacrificed your own happiness over and over again to try to show him how much you care.

Although there is a part of you that wants to leave, the team senses that you could not live with yourself if you had not convinced yourself that you had done everything in your power to demonstrate the depth of your love for him. From what you have told us about him, he is a man who may feel unlovable, in spite of your attempts to show your love for him. You also know that you are the only woman who may ever convince him that he could be loved, and that you fear what would become of him if you were to leave him. We are sorry to say that we see no easy way out of this situation for you. We are afraid that in order to convince him of your love, you may have to make the ultimate sacrifice for him. You may have to stand in front of his loaded gun and let him pull the trigger so that he will understand that you love him so much you would be willing to give up your life to prove your love for him.

(pp. 230–231)

We scheduled a follow-up visit with her. She assured us that she would be safe until then, and we could count on seeing her. A couple of days later, she returned for the scheduled follow-up visit. We told her that we had been worried that her situation might have deteriorated since her previous visit. She smiled and said:

I don't know why, but on the way home I started thinking about what you said last time. When I got home, I went up to him and asked if his gun was still out in the truck. He said it was, and I asked him if it was loaded. He said no, so I told him to get it, load it, and come back in and shoot me because I wasn't going to spend the rest of my life trying to convince him that I loved him and worrying about whether he believed me. He wouldn't get the gun. I think he was surprised that I stood up for myself. Anyway, things have been different for the last few days.

(p. 231)

Sharon's creative solution to her own problem was completely unpredictable. As I speculated in the original article, "The position taken by the therapy team was one which apparently was congruent with the client's world view, did not arouse resistance, and enabled the client to act differently because she thought differently about her situation" (p. 231). In the follow-up session, Sharon described the household as being peaceful, and that Jerry seemed to be more loving and attentive. However, she also recognized that his change of heart was one she had seen before after a violent episode. So, she, and we, were only cautiously optimistic. We suggested to Sharon that she might now take advantage of the shifting winds and bring Jerry in for a couple's session. She said that she had already asked him to come with her and that he had been planning to come with her, but she thought she should run the idea by us first. We enthusiastically endorsed her plan. She and Jerry arrived a few days later for a conjoint session where we began to work with Jerry and Sharon to improve their relationship.

Our understanding of this case considered the contributions of second-order cybernetics thinking (Griffith, Griffith, & Slovik, 1990). We understood that the reality of the problem was linguistically created by everyone who was in a relationship with the problem, including the clients, the therapists and the team members. That is, we endeavored to include ourselves in the formulation of the case. Almost every other helper/advice-giver had attempted to separate the couple. Some of these attempts were overt, such as encouraging her to leave him, sheltering her in a half-way house, and so on. Others were more covert, such as encouraging her to improve her self-esteem and standing on her own two feet. For us, it might have been considered unethical to suggest the same options that had already been tried and failed.[7] Our approach was not only an intervention into Sharon and Jerry's interactions, but their interactions with other help-givers, and even their interactions with us. We knew that at that point in an extremely volatile situation, we wanted to avoid prescribing more of the same.

Example 4: The Angry Teenager

The second case I described in that 1987 *JMFT* paper was the last I saw as a Fellow at GFI before I left for a full-time job at Our Lady of the Lake University. Once a week, GFI had an afternoon training group that met in Houston. I was one of the co-supervisors in the group. One of the participants in the group, who worked for the juvenile probation department, requested a consultation interview with one of her teenage clients, Marie. The probation department was considering placing 16-year-old Marie in a half-way house but were concerned about recent threats that she had made against Mrs. Thompson, whom she felt was responsible for the death of Marie's baby. The probation officer asked me a week earlier to provide the therapy and told me that he had already asked Marie if she would be willing to meet with me to discuss her situation. He brought her to the interview and she had no objections to his observing the session from behind the one-way mirror.

I started the interview by briefly asking about the solutions that Marie had attempted or considered. Those might have been viewed as members of the class of solutions that she'd attempted and failed at or rejected. Notice that the following elaboration of this reframing was done within Marie's worldview.

Monte: The thing that I'm impressed with is that you thought about a lot of ways to even the score with Mrs. Thompson. You thought about pushing her down the stairs, about shooting her, putting out a contract on her, and suing her… I'm just amazed that as angry as you are you're willing to let her off so easy.

Marie: (*looking up surprised*) What do you mean "let her off easy"?

Monte: Well, you said that she was real scared... And that you could already see that it was on her conscience... that she already feels pretty guilty about it... (*Marie resumes staring at her feet.*)

Marie: And, she is!

Monte: ... and a woman like that is likely to have that on her mind for the rest of her life and is probably not going to be able to sleep very well at night. She will probably be a miserable, sad old woman for the rest of her life because of that... But, ... If you go ahead and kill her next week, that's letting her off easy because she won't have to suffer very long. You might do her a big favor by killing her... I guess I don't understand why you would be willing to let her off so easy, because if you kill her it will be over, like that (*snaps fingers*). And she won't have to suffer.

(p. 234)

Comment: This further elaboration begins to suggest an alternative meaning for Mrs. Thompson's death – relief from suffering – that was not the one that Marie was attempting to communicate by her revenge. When I said that Marie would do Mrs. Thompson a big favor by killing her, it was because Marie was not at all interested in doing Mrs. Thompson any favors. Here I was capitalizing on Marie's anger and uncharitable feelings toward Mrs. Thompson.

Marie: (*looking up*) So, what you're saying is just let her suffer?

Monte: Well, I just wonder which would be worse for her. To live for the next 50 years with the death of your baby on her conscience day and night or if you were just to put her out of her misery?

Marie: (*30-second pause, looking down*) I don't know, because I'm very angry.

Monte: (*after a phoned suggestion from the team*) ... You know, you were talking about showing her a picture of your baby. (*Client looks up again*) I think even that would be letting her off easy. You should *give* her a picture of your baby, ... If you don't decide to let her off real easy.

Marie: Give her *my* baby's pictures? (*Incredulous*)

Monte: You could make copies for her. So that she'll be reminded every day while she's in that place with all those pregnant women, about what she did... killing her would certainly make *you* feel better, but it would be letting *her* off easy... if she were to die next week, *you* would still have *your* baby on *your* mind for the rest of *your* life, and you're going to be suffering for the rest of your life with the memory of what happened. It'll probably keep you up at night sometimes... Of course, if you or your Bandito friends [a well-known motorcycle gang that Marie claimed to have connections with] kill her, she wouldn't be suffering the same way you're going to continue to suffer.

Comment: Here I was trying to frame, more explicitly, that killing Mrs. Thompson could have a different meaning than simple revenge, if one considers that part of Marie's thinking is that not only she, but other people, needed to see that her baby's death has been avenged. The meaning being offered creates some doubt as to whether murder will accomplish her goals. I was also trying to speak Marie's language of self-sacrifice here.

Marie: … Sounds like a good idea, giving her a picture of my baby *(looks up, smiling).*

Comment: Here Marie acknowledged that the suggested solution had more potential to achieve her goals than the previous course of action she had considered.

Monte: … Well, you need to give some careful consideration and thought to what you want to do, because it may be that you want to let her off the easy way…

Comment: Here again, I am taking advantage of Marie's unwillingness to be at all kind to Mrs. Thompson.

Marie: (60-second pause, looks up) Where can I get copies made?

(pp. 234–235)

Comment: At this point, I could hear muffled cheers coming from the observation room as the team recognized that the case had turned a corner. No need for a follow-up appointment was seen. The probation officer who had referred her was behind the mirror and confident that Marie would not be a threat to Mrs. Thompson. Plans were already in the making to have Marie transfer to a different living situation, because she was no longer pregnant. Later, we were able to follow up with the probation officer who had referred Marie to us. The officer escorted Marie, at her request, to a photo finishing store where Marie had copies made of her baby's pictures. She proudly gave one to Mrs. Thompson before she was placed in another half-way house. Reportedly, Mrs. Thompson thanked her for the photo and no angry words were exchanged.

Example 5: Harry on the Hotline

In the early 1990s, Harry Goolishian was giving a workshop on brief family therapy at Our Lady of the Lake University in San Antonio. Toward the end of the day, one of the participants presented the common challenge about how to use brief therapy with clients that may be talking about suicide. Harry told the following story[8]:

Let me give you an example. This is a story some of you have heard.

Before I retired from the Medical School, one of the benefits of being on the faculty there was that you got to staff the emergency room one night a month. *(audience laughter)* It was always a harrowing and tiring experience.

It was about 11 o'clock at night, and the nurse handed me the telephone and said, "Dr. Goolishian. You'd better take this."

And I said, "All right, Psychiatric Emergency Room." And someone said, in a deep and sonorous voice, "Can you use my body?" *(audience laughter)* It was a male voice. And, this was a couple of years ago, so my memory is a little sketchy, but basically what I said, immediately in return was, "I don't know. Is it useful?" They asked me a direct question, "Can you use my body"? and I give him a direct answer: "'I don't know. Is it useful?"

And the guy said, "Of course it's useful! Aren't you guys doing some research down there?" and one thing and another.

Harry: "We're doing all sorts of research, and whether your body is useful or not would depend on how you intend to kill yourself. Because some types of suicide would make your body not useful in our research."

And he said, "Oh." What else is he gonna say? *(audience chuckles)*

And, uh, one thing led to another, and he started talking about the fact that he was from Dallas.

Harry: "Oh, you're in Dallas?"

And he said, "Yeah."

Harry: "You know, this is Galveston. How come you don't give your body to somebody up there?"

And then he went on and told this long story about how the people up there were no good, and pushed him around, and had used him, and one thing and another . . . And, I sat thinking, "Oh, that's useful information."

Harry: "You know, you're really putting me on the spot."

Caller: "How's that?"

Harry: "This is the night clinic, you got."

Caller: "I know it's the night time!"

Harry: You know, I've been trying hard to get on the day clinic. And, the reason I'm on the night clinic is: The Dean doesn't think I am good enough to be on the day clinic. And, if I sent an ambulance all the way up to Dallas to get your body, and it wasn't useful for our research, I'd be on the night clinic the rest of my life!

And this guy had been pushed around by authority enough, and he knew exactly … and, began to be very sympathetic and supportive. And, he began doing therapy with me! Trying to reassure me that someday I'd make it. And, just stick in there … And, that went on for a while, finally we got back down to the basic issue about whether or not we wanted his body. And, I asked,

Harry: "How are you gonna kill yourself?"

And, he said he was going to take, I think, it was strychnine, I can't remember, but I think it was strychnine.

Harry: "Oh my god. That's another tough one."

Caller: "How's that?"

Harry: "Well, that's one of the courses I didn't do too well in in school."

Caller: "What do you mean?"

Harry: "I don't know what that would do to your body. We're doing some very delicate eye research, and that might make your eyes not useful."

Caller: "Well, how you gonna find out?!"

Harry: "Well, I'll have to ask the pharmacologist. I simply don't know the answer to that. As I said, I flunked that course."

The caller said, "Oh, you're going to call the police," and one thing and another.

Harry: "I don't blame you for believing that because ordinarily, that would be the thing to do, and I know I can't reassure you. I'm really puzzled now. I'm not sure how to do this. How we're going to solve this problem."

And, we argued about that for a while, and it became very clear that unless he told me where he was calling from, I couldn't get the information he wanted. And, he wasn't going to give me the information because I'd call the police … and, I just became even more inept about knowing what to do. And, finally, in desperation, he said, "Oh, dammit! Call the pharmacologist!" And he gave me his phone number.

And, I waited about 15 minutes and called him back. And the first ring, bang, like that.

Caller: "What did you find out?"

Harry: "Well, we're in real trouble."

Caller: "How's that??"

Harry: "Arsenic is going to ruin your eyes for this research."

Caller: "Arsenic??"

Harry: "Yeah, isn't that what you're going to use?"

Caller: "You dumb son of a bitch! I told you it was strychnine! Don't you get anything right?"

And, uh, then he went on and berated me about how I'd be on the night clinic the rest of my life. I deserved to be on the night clinic. I couldn't keep anything straight, and just really chewed me out. And, I just kept apologizing, forgetting, and I took a real one-down. And he became real kind to me, and supportive to me, and he didn't mean to be so mad at me, and that it was important to him that his body be used, and I agreed. That I didn't know how he was going to do it. That I had fouled it up and had probably messed his life up.

And, finally in desperation, he said, "Would you do me a favor?"

Harry: "Yeah."

Caller: "Would you call the cops, and have them bring me to the hospital?"

And I did, and they did, and he didn't kill himself. It took about an hour.

This story was classic Harry. Behind the humor this story evokes is a subtle humanitarian ethos that represented Harry's work. Harry never failed to be struck by the irony of the situations we find ourselves in. Often taking a step back, as he did, allowed that irony to manifest itself. The years I spent studying and following Harry around, our endless late-night discussions in bars and fishing on the end of Harry's dock (Bobele, 2003), taught me the value of looking past the obvious. One evening while I was unsuccessfully fishing for flounder on his dock, Harry told me that the secret was knowing when the fish had swallowed the bait.

> "Well, Harry," I started, "how do you tell the difference between the tug that he makes from just sucking it in, and the tug on the line that comes from when he swallows the bait?"
>
> "When you figure that out," he began with a mischievous smile and an index finger in the air, "you'll be able to catch more flounder."
>
> With that, he turned and headed back up the dock to the house. As I watched him go, I could not help feeling that I had just learned something about fishing *and* working with clients.
>
> (Bobele, 2003, p. 5)

In this case, it is notable that the "suicidal" client called a hospital 300 miles way and was charitable enough to be an organ donor. We might speculate on whether Harry picked up on the subtle ambivalence. I think he did. He was an excellent fisherman.

Looking Backwards and Forwards

As I continued to study and practice, guided by Harry and other mentors, I found myself beginning to think my more conventionally trained peers were actually working paradoxically. I began to understand that the meaning of paradox for many of them was an intervention (a *You Said What?*) that occurred when one therapist said or did something that did not fit within the observer's worldview. For example, Erickson's instructions to insomniacs to remain awake and stay awake runs counter to the idea that one should count sheep (bore oneself), exercise (tire oneself), do relaxation exercises (calm oneself), and so on. I found myself seeing that other therapists were practicing paradoxically, from my perspective.

A client arrives at the therapist's office in a crisis and is told they have to make an appointment, complete numerous forms, assessments, and wait a long time for the therapy to have an effect – that seems paradoxical to me. Forms of therapy, like psychoanalysis, that discourage talk about the immediate concerns of the client in favor of other, "deeper," hidden meanings strike me as paradoxical (see Haley, 1969). I found that these new, outside-of-the-box, non-linear, postmodern, post-structural, social constructionist ways of thinking began to permeate the ways I thought about the dilemmas clients bring to us. These ways of thinking began to shape my appreciation for the counter-dilemmas (to rephrase the Milan team's *counter-paradox*) we offered to clients.

When I look back on the work reported here, I can't help but think that I would do things differently today. Frankly, I think many of us took some pride in coming up with clever, unusual interventions to use. I don't think we have moved away from that urge completely. Some therapists pride themselves on the clever, unusual letters and ceremonies that they create. Others, from a position of "evidence-based practice," develop highly structured, manualized treatment programs without regard to the idiosyncrasies of clients. I think, for me, I have moved away from thinking that my expertise lies in being provocative, as Haley and Erickson were, to being more modest in my expectations. I have come to respect clients' own wisdom in knowing what is best for them. I now frequently ask clients, "If I were to give you a useful homework assignment," or "If I were to give you some really good advice," what would it be?[9]

Part of the move, for me, away from the heavy-handed instrumentalism of MRI and the Milan group, was the growing recognition that a more collaborative, non-hierarchical position with clients was emerging as a therapeutic position in the field. The evolution of the GFI/HGI's non-expert position (Anderson & Goolishian, 1992) was a valuable contribution to how we thought of ourselves in relationship to our clients and was important in shaping my softening of the way I thought of intervening in people's lives. The importance of the mutual influence became more important than sharpening our interventive skills when working with clients. I think the times have changed, we have moved to more contextual ways of viewing our roles as therapists. When I look back at some of the cases I worked with years ago, I can see the clients' expertise shining through. Harry used to say that several years after he had seen a client, he hoped he would be so insignificant that clients would have forgotten his name. If anything, they would remember him as a kind man who was fumbling to be helpful, but the clients had found their own solutions before he could get around to it. For any therapist, that is a worthy goal.

Notes

1 One sign of the innovative, cutting-edge atmosphere in Galveston in those days was the publication of *Multiple Impact Therapy* by MacGregor et al. in 1964, the same year as Satir's *Conjoint Family Therapy* (1964). It is generally accepted that these were the first two books published that were entirely devoted to family therapy. Of the MIT book, Satir (1965) said in her review, "I believe that this book may well become a classic among studies on families and family therapy."
2 I am grateful to Paul Dell for his permission to use this material.
3 Rob graciously reviewed this account and gave permission for its publication.
4 This case was extremely complex and the complete rationale for the intervention matches that complexity. Interested readers are referred to the original paper in *JMFT*.
5 As a training institute, GFI used a model that had therapists in the consultation room interviewing the client(s), while the rest of the team observed from behind a one-way mirror.
6 The page numbers following the quotations in these two cases are from the original 1987 article.
7 Again, the reader is referred to Bobele (1987, 1988), Woody and Woody (1988), and Weakland (1988) for further discussion; as well as to pp. 215–216 in our Editors' Conclusion (Chapter 20 this volume).
8 Fortunately, we videotaped the presentation. The following is from the transcript.
9 Some might point out that such questions are paradoxical in that the therapist is asking the client for advice rather than the other way around!

References

Anderson, H., & Goolishian, H.A. (1992). The client is the expert: A not-knowing approach to therapy. In S. McNamee & K.J. Gergen (Eds.), *Therapy as social construction* (pp. 25–39). Newbury Park, CA: Sage.

Bateson, G. (1972). *Steps to an ecology of mind*. San Francisco: Chandler Publishing Company.

Bobele, M. (1987). Therapeutic interventions in life-threatening situations. *Journal of Marriage and Family Therapy, 13*(3), 225–239.

Bobele, M. (1989). Interactional treatment of intractable hiccups. *Family Process, 28,* 191–206.

Bobele, M. (1988). 'Public policy in life-threatening situations': Reply. *Journal of Marital And Family Therapy, 14*(2), 139–141. doi:10.1111/j.1752-0606.1988.tb00729.x

Bobele, M. (2003). Floundering with Harry. *Journal of The Texas Association for Marriage and Family Therapy, 8*(1), 4–5.

Duvall, J., Carleton, D., & Tremblay, C. (2015). Reengaging history with Harlene Anderson: Nosey Rosie Goes! Part I. *Journal of Systemic Therapies, 34*(4), 61–79. http://doi.org/10.1521/jsyt.2015.34.4.61

Duvall, J., Carleton, D., & Tremblay, C. (2016). Reengaging history with Harlene Anderson: Nosey RosieGoes! Part II. *Journal of Systemic Therapies, 35*(1), 61–77. http://doi.org/10.1521/jsyt.2016.35.1.61

Griffith, J., Griffith, M., Slovik, L. (1990). Mind-body problems in family therapy: Contrasting first- and second-order cybernetics approaches. *Family Process, 29*(1), 13–28.

Haley, J. (1969). *The power tactics of Jesus Christ, and other essays.* New York: Avon.

Haley, J. (1971). *Advanced techniques of hypnosis and therapy.* New York: Grune & Stratton.

Haley, J. (1973). *Uncommon therapy: The psychiatric techniques of Milton H. Erickson, M.D.* New York: Norton.

MacGregor, R., Ritchie, A. M., Serrano, A. C., Schuster, F. (1964). *Multiple impact therapy with families.* New York: McGraw-Hill.

Palazzoli, M.S., Cecchin, G., Prata, G., & Boscolo, L. (1978). *Paradox and counterparadox: A new model in the therapy of the family in schizophrenic transaction.* New York: Aronson.

Ruesch, J., & Bateson, G. (1951). *Communication: The social matrix of psychiatry.* New York: Norton.

Satir, V. M. (1964). *Conjoint family therapy.* Palo Alto, CA: Science and Behavior Books.

Satir, V. M. (1965). *Review of Multiple Impact Therapy with Families. American Journal of Orthopsychiatry, 35*(1), 173–174. doi:10.1037/h0097069

Watzlawick, P. (1983). *The situation is hopeless but not serious.* New York: Norton.

Watzlawick, P., Weakland, J. H., & Fisch, R. (1974). *Change: Principles of problem formation and problem resolution.* New York: Norton.

Weakland, J. H., Fisch, R., Watzlawick, P., & Bodin, A. (1974). Brief therapy: Focused problem resolution. *Family Process, 13,* 146–159.

Weakland, J. H. (1988). Weakland on the Woodys-Bobele exchange. *Journal of Marital and Family Therapy, 14*(2), 205.

Woody, J. D. (1990). Resolving ethical concerns in clinical practice: Toward a pragmatic model. *Journal of Marital and Family Therapy, 16*(2), 133–150. doi:10.1111/j.1752-0606.1990.tb00834.x

Woody, J. D., & Woody, R. H. (1988). Public policy in life-threatening situations: A response to Bobele. *Journal of Marital and Family Therapy, 14*(2), 133–137.

CHAPTER 5

A Violent Life[1]
Using Brief Therapy "Logics" to Facilitate Change

Flavio Cannistrá

When the ward's headmistress introduced me to Daniel, I was looking at an ageless young man: he could have been 30 as well as 50. He dressed like a "b-boy" (a hip-hop rapper or street break-dancer): oversized, ragged trousers and T-shirt, worn-out windbreaker, shabby cap. But the deep dark circles under his eyes, a leathery, hardened skin, the strong odor of someone who hadn't had a shower in days and the lack of most of his teeth gave his figure an aged look.

I held out my hand, and he gave me a contemptuous look without even trying to hide it. He slightly shook it, looking away. When we sat in our room, for some reason, the first thing I asked him was: "How are you doing?" And he unambiguously answered, "Shitty."

Context

Daniel was in the Mental Hygiene Center where I did my internship and trained for three and a half years. It is located in a rough district on the outskirts of Rome, far from where tourists go. All our meetings occurred in Italian. Each week, I saw individuals and couples, usually from the lower middle class, about the most diverse issues: anxiety and mood disorders, personality disorders, and even marriage conflicts and relational disorders.

My work with Daniel was very interesting and surprising. He was clearly violent. He had a justified distrust toward doctors and therapists. His story was one full of dark corners. Nonetheless, starting with a couple of simple strategies, he and I succeeded in unblocking an invalidating problem and opened a therapeutic path that invested his whole personality. In this chapter, I will describe the techniques I used with Daniel. I will also elaborate a system that I have been developing the last few years that helps me to identify the best techniques to use with my patients. I will alternate narrative sections with theoretical descriptions that will help the reader understand my strategies and therapeutic choices.

First Session

Daniel came from a small town in Sicily, neck-deep in a depressed social-economic environment. His first encounter with the Mental Hygiene Services (MHS) was the one that scarred him for the next two-and-a-half decades of his life. At ten, his exuberant and antagonistic personality was tamed in a radical and questionable way: he was stuffed with massive quantities of psychopharmaceuticals. In the following 25 years (Daniel was 34 when we met – "Just three years older than me!?" I thought), the situation had plummeted. He brawled, participated in the criminal underground, went in and out of the MHS, was sometimes forcibly hospitalized, and even went through a time in prison. And then, "for the last time," Daniel decided to turn to a Mental Hygiene Center.

I'm a licensed psychologist and psychotherapist. At the time I worked with Daniel, my main field was Brief Strategic Therapy, an approach that I studied at the Center for Strategic Therapy in Arezzo, Italy (Nardone & Watzlawick, 1993). Although I have since studied different kinds of brief therapy and had received a master's degree in Ericksonian hypnosis from the Italian Hypnosis Society, and have studied Single-Session Therapy with Michael Hoyt in California and at the Bouverie Centre in Australia (after which I founded the Italian Center for Single Session Therapy – see Cannistrá & Piccirilli, 2018), at that time I had just begun my specialization in Brief Strategic Therapy. Hence, that was the main approach I chose for the case, although other influences naturally played a part in my work with Daniel.

Defining the Aim

One of the traits in common among brief therapies is the quick definition of a therapeutic goal (Budman, Hoyt, & Friedman, 1992; Hoyt, 2009). When you work in the here-and-now, it is essential to identify a concrete goal mutually agreed upon with the patient, instead of focusing on a long study of the patient's history or their unconscious dynamics. Setting a goal helps to build a solid therapeutic alliance. But, when I tried to define the goal with Daniel, just after being told that he was doing "shitty," I hadn't imagined the burden I was going to take.

"Why 'shitty'?" I asked.

"Doctor … Lil' Doc. Can I call you Lil' Doc?" – he grinned – "The problem is I like to beat the shit out of people." He stopped, weighing and evaluating the effect that his words had had on me. Something moved in my stomach. I finally had a word for the feeling I had been having – *fear*. "Am I in front of a dangerous person?" I wondered.

I tried to act authoritative and, following my studies of Solution-Focused Brief Therapy (SFBT; de Shazer, 1988; O'Connell, 2012), I tried to identify a possible exception to the problem to better understand how it worked:

"Elaborate on that – you like it before or after a fight?" I asked.

Daniel was surprised. Why didn't this doctor just tell him that fighting is wrong, and that he should have been ashamed of himself like the other doctors had? But his wonder lasted just a few seconds, hidden behind another grin. "I like it before, when I sense fear in their eyes. I like it throughout, when I feel my knuckles break their faces. And, I like it after, when I see them lying on the ground in a pool of blood."

These were his words. He was provoking me. Later on, some colleagues told me that Daniel clearly had a histrionic personality. Maybe so, but I wasn't interested in labels, and that didn't change the important fact that Daniel *did* beat people up.

"Why should this be a problem?" I asked Daniel. For myself, I can imagine how it's a problem taking pleasure in "beating the shit out of people" but, according to radical constructivist thought (Watzlawick, 1984), it is of great importance to identify the *other* person's point of view in order to achieve therapeutic success. Since, as Hoyt (2017, p. xiii) said, "How you look influences what you see, and what you see influences what you do," the danger of looking through *my* lenses, and not through the client's, is always around the corner. Although Heinz von Foerster (1984) masterfully proved that it is impossible to completely escape our own point of view, the account given by the other is still, in the end, *our* interpretation of the facts. It is, of course, possible to make our subjectivity recede, leaving as much room as possible for the patient's interpretation. The patient's therapeutic aim, then, not ours, becomes easier to achieve. That is why I needed to know why, *in his opinion*, beating the shit out of people was a problem.

"Just Three Sessions"

Years earlier, my older colleague, Dr. Paola Lancia, referred to me a patient with a troublesome drinking problem. I didn't want to give up on that case, but I didn't know if I was able to handle it. So, I applied a strategy that my colleague suggested. I offered to do no more than three sessions, at the end of which we would be able to judge what we had done and decide if we still had to go on. (That therapy lasted for 27 sessions, and it was a complete success.) With Daniel, I applied the same method, especially after I heard the urgent reason that had compelled him to look for a psychologist again.

"Why is it a problem?" he repeated. "Lil' Doc, a year ago I came out of prison. I was there two years of my life. I know how it is, I know what is waiting for me, and I can't go there again. But, if I keep on beating people up, sooner or later they are going to bust me again. And next time it won't be for just two years. If something like this should happen again, next time *I won't stand it*."

As much as his ways were theatrical, the possibility he mentioned was real. Punching people was a good way to go to jail, especially if you were an ex-convict who had been jailed for the same reason before. This problem was compounded by the fact that in prison, the pleasure of "beating people to death" wasn't going to disappear. At that moment, I felt all the weight of the case: If I didn't help Daniel manage his problem, he would risk getting involved in a brawl each and every single day. He could end up in prison again and, once there, he would meet his grim end. I was facing a real predicament.

Using an analogy from Fisch et al. (1982), Daniel seemed like one of those window shoppers who take a stroll and, when it unexpectedly starts to rain, enters a shop without any intention of buying anything. Actually, according to SFBT's outlook, Daniel really looked like a *customer* (O'Connell, 2012), someone who is aware that he has a problem and wants to do everything that is necessary to solve it. But, from a pragmatic-communicative point of view, he tended to establish one-up complementary interactions (Watzlawick, Beavin & Jackson, 1967): he wanted to lead, and the danger of creating a symmetry was really great. How would he react if he felt I was challenging him? So, I decided from the beginning to take a one-down position, as John Weakland teaches (Green, 1995), and I proposed the three sessions to him – as will be illustrated in what follows. Before doing so, however, I needed to have his complete trust.

Speaking the Client's Language

There was something I knew while I was speaking with Daniel. In spite of what he had said, he didn't really "like" to beat the shit out of people. His reaction was an explosive aggressiveness. He more or less always insulted whomever he thought was giving him a bad look – something that could happen with anyone and at any time. If that person answered back, everything would end up in a physical clash. The question was not *if* Daniel would fight again, but rather *when* it would happen. I understood that quickly enough during the first session, and I immediately thought about how to disarm it. However, I was not sure that I could do it. First of all, I had to win his confidence.

If I were asked to pick up only one useful idea from Milton Erickson, I would choose "speak your client's language" without any doubt. Erickson referred mainly to the need to meet the person using the way the person perceives the world and gives meanings, instead of making the patient adhere to our theory (Watzlawick, 1978). In my opinion, this advice can be taken too literally by someone who thinks it is all about using the client's "words." On this occasion, however, I had the strong feeling that the very words I used in the session's closing section had had a great impact on our relation and on the therapy as a whole.

After some 40 minutes spent defining his problem and the way it worked, I took a moment to reflect and looked out of the window. Still not looking at him, I said: *"You are right, you know"* – I paused before looking him straight in the eyes – *"it really is shitty."*

Daniel's expression changed, as if to say *"What, you heard me? Did you just agree?"* He set his intense, half-closed blue eyes on me, eyebrows plunged into a confused frown, and for the very first time never took them away again.

He looked as though he was pondering, *"Why don't you lecture me?"* He was offering me all his attention. I kept on thinking that I had to acknowledge the seriousness of his problem, the fact that, if no doctor had helped him in the last 25 years – on the contrary, they had worsened his situation – a "young doctor" like me couldn't be sure to be of any help. So, I proposed the three-sessions idea to set a limited number of meetings and see what the result was going to be. Daniel didn't understand it right then, and, emerging from the deep-attention state he was in, he smashed his fist down on the table, *"Do you really think you can heal me in three sessions?!"*

I froze, keeping my temper: "I'm sorry, I didn't mean that." I had inadvertently underplayed years of suffering, pharmaceuticals, psychiatric examinations, and jail time. I tried to mend the situation: "Of course we're not going to make it in three sessions. I'm sure that within three sessions we aren't going to achieve anything. What I mean is that after three sessions we are going to evaluate the status of the situation. If we are both satisfied, we go on; if not, we stop. I don't want to waste your time."

He looked at me for some time, as to understand whether I wanted to fool him. And then he said: *"All right."*

First Session Tasks

To me, it was clear that Daniel's problem was the way he perceived others, but I didn't think it was wise to work on that from the very beginning. I asked him instead to identify the "risky" situations during the next week, so that I could better understand how they worked: "From here to the next session, please take note of all the situations that might be risky, that could bring you to lose your patience – or, in other words, to punch someone." I wanted him to observe the situations that could put him in a condition to fight people.[2]

Actually, the main aim was to strengthen our relationship. I was in the process of choosing the most apt techniques to use, the ones that I would have improved on only later (I will elaborate more on this below), but I was sure that, on this occasion, the first step to make was to strengthen our relationship with a task that would show my interest in his problem.

The Nine Logics Beneath Brief Therapy Interventions

Hundreds of brief therapy techniques exist. We can trace their origins to at least four main sources: Milton Erickson's (1967, 1980) work, the MRI Brief Therapy Center's model (Fisch et al., 1982; Watzlawick et al., 1974), Solution-Focused Brief Therapy (de Shazer, 1988; de Shazer, Dolan, Korman, Trepper, MacCollum & Berg, 2006), and, of course, Arezzo's Brief Strategic Therapy (Nardone & Watzlawick, 1993).

The great variety of *techniques*, however, does not correspond to an equivalent number of *logics of intervention*. With a specific *effect* or *objective* in mind (e.g., reducing a manifestation of anxiety), the therapist follows a certain *logic* or *purpose* (e.g., blocking a certain behavior), and to do that therapists use one or more *techniques*. Similar to the relationship between *strategy* and *tactics*, interventions or maneuvers could be different in form but obey the same logic. Using that same logic, the therapist chooses the technique or specific intervention that is considered most likely to be effective for that particular person and situation. When the logic is identified, it is easier to adapt, change, or even invent a new technique, since the logic beneath it is clear.

The full panoply of techniques I have reviewed are discussed in detail elsewhere (Cannistrá, 2018), together with bibliography, methodology, and examples. Here I will just briefly identify nine logics[3].

1 **Direct block of attempted solution:** This logic includes those techniques which call in a more or less direct way for the patient to stop a certain behavior in order to block the attempted solution[4].
2 **Create aversion:** This logic includes those techniques aimed at creating in the patient an aversion toward something, such as a behavior, or a form of interaction or relationship, etc.
3 **Creating awareness:** This series of techniques are meant to help the client become aware of something, such as a wrong behavior or misperception of their abilities and resources.
4 **Create from seemingly nothing:** This logic includes techniques that are designed to introduce changes (small or large) in clients' perceptions and behaviors in order to create or amplify resources, skills and abilities.
5 **Increase to reduce:** Within this category is a large number of paradoxical techniques.
6 **Small changes (or small violations):** This logic includes those techniques aimed at solving a problem by implementing small, often incremental, changes. "Go slow!" John Weakland would often advise to avoid stimulating resistance; Erickson would use *partitioning* to break down problems into smaller parts and *progression* to build on a series of small gains (Short et al., 2005).
7 **Strengthen the relationship:** Essentially designed to strengthen the therapeutic alliance, this is the only one of the nine logics that is not intended to *directly* produce a therapeutic result. As common factors researchers (e.g., Duncan et al., 2010) have shown, this accounts for about 30% of the variance in change.
8 **Shift the focus:** Many techniques can be designed to shift the patient's attention, thus distracting them from perceptions and behaviors that would continue a problem.
9 **Express and process:** The last category includes all those techniques that aim to vent and/or further process a particular lived experience and thus may lead to feelings of a different kind.

We need to remember that a technique is merely an instrument obeying the logic of intervention. When facing challenging situations, once the logic is identified ("What specifically am I trying to accomplish right now?") the therapist can select and employ appropriate techniques.

Let us now go back to Daniel and see how I put into practice some of these ideas.

Second Session

Daniel came back the following week. He had done the task necessary to *strengthen our relationship (Logic #7)*: I thought that it was a positive result because he had done what I had requested to help me understand him more. He described some situations to me – such as a time when he got pissed off because a co-worker had asked him to work a little faster – that confirmed my hypothesis that the main issue was Daniel's constant perception of hostility and menace from others, to which he responded with aggressiveness and violence. A traditional medical-psychiatric vocabulary would have defined him as having a Paranoid Personality Disorder. The problem was that Daniel didn't realize that he perceived what he thought people were thinking about him, and not their real attitude toward him. I wanted to block this perception and, at the same time, make him conscious of the bias.

According to the logics I have identified, increasing the problematic behavior of Daniel perceiving threats (*#5, Increase to reduce*) would help to make him aware of his behavior (*#3, Creating awareness*). I remembered a paradoxical technique that I had learned in my studies for similar situations: *the search for confirmation* (for in-depth analyses of paradoxical techniques, see Weeks, 2012; Weeks & L'Abate, 1982; Fisch et al., 1982; Watzlawick et al., 1974). The clients are asked to actively seek, every day, signs on the faces of other people that confirm they have something against them. Although it may look like a dangerous technique, it really isn't (unless the person is showing severe psychotic symptoms). Whoever thinks that someone else is threatening or holding a grudge, just *thinks* it: "A suspicious person is a person who has something on his mind. He looks at the world with fixed and preoccupying expectation, and he searches repetitively, and only, for confirmation of it" (Shapiro, 1965, p. 56).

Moreover, in a vicious circle, right when the person observes someone with the idea of being threatened or mocked, the client will probably respond with a challenging look and attitude, making the other act ... actually threatening or hostile! It is a classic example of a *self-fulfilling prophecy* (Watzlawick et al., 1967). When we ask the client to actively look for specific signs of threat or hostility, when we encourage a client to look from outside of his or her own thought and use their ability to minutely analyze reality, the patient may not use a global, challenging approach anymore, and, more important, may not look for *confirmation*, but for *hints* instead. The client will not take for granted that the other is threatening/hostile. For the first time, the person may look at a face in an active, aware way, for objective signs of menace. And, of course, these are almost always nowhere to be found.

This is exactly what happened with Daniel.

Third Session

When Daniel came back the third week, he was annoyed. I investigated the results of the task, and he had the answer I was waiting for: There were no signs of hostility from the people that he met on those days. The first case he reported to me that week was about a young man whose face he had studied at the bus stop. Daniel reported: "He looked at me and I said, 'What the f**k you looking at?!' and then he immediately lowered his eyes." Daniel grinned.

"OK, I understand. Tell me, as you were looking at him, did you identify which were the signs that confirmed that he held something against you?"

Daniel looked away: "There were none. He had nothing to do with me."

"Nothing to do with you?"

"No – there was nothing. I have to say, he did not do anything – but he was still a jerk."

During his life, Daniel had built his whole personality around this problem. We had created a fissure, an opening in his previously hermetically sealed worldview.

Following Sessions

The work with Daniel lasted for a year and a half; one session per week. Although surliness and irreverence were part of his personality, the feelings of being threatened or mocked by others disappeared within the first three sessions. By our fourth meeting, I didn't need to tell him to apply the *search for confirmation*. He had realized that it was him who was seeing hostility in the eyes of the others. I mostly limited myself to *reframing* interventions[5] that asked him to describe and examine evidence that others were threatening him, in order to help him understand that a series of events where he had perceived a provocation could be attributed to a misinterpretation of his, or to his provocation (*#3, Creating awareness*). Through the previous decades, Daniel had developed a provocative disposition, dotted with a challenging and hostile attitude toward other people. That was the problem that took the longest to resolve. First, we worked on the immense anger he felt, caused by a life spent with people and in places that he had survived only through fighting. His anger was mainly directed toward "fate," toward his financial situation, toward the place he lived (a dilapidated building where rain leaked in and wind swept through the cracks in the wall), toward his past full of brawls, drugs and loneliness, but above all, toward the people who hadn't found a better way to cure him than to feed him pharmaceuticals and label him as an antisocial type, a basket case.

I knew that a way to reduce anger is often to write it down (Patrick, 2013; Pennebaker, 1997; Pennebaker & Beall, 1986), but I realized that it wasn't possible with Daniel. Because he had left school after primary school, writing was a great effort for him, and an embarrassing one. He usually brought back small pieces of paper with five or six lines written on them that didn't achieve any therapeutic effect. But, he had a talent. He could really draw well. Since the logic stayed the same (*#9, Express and process*), I adapted the technique to this talent. I once asked him to draw what he felt, and he poured forth all his anger. The effect was quick enough, and within a few sessions his anger lowered considerably, and he eventually learned to do it on his own, drawing when he wanted to unload.

In subsequent sessions, we often discussed how to relate with others and what kinds of emotional and behavioral reactions he could create with his behaviors. Once again, the logic I often followed was to *create awareness*. This gave him a different, less volatile sense of power and control. Over time, Daniel's arrogant and annoying personality smoothed. I never had the illusion that he would turn out "a good boy," but he changed enough to alter his attitude when he was at work, where in spite of often being irritated and sometimes irritating, he succeeded in keeping a job as a cook in a small café for almost a year. At the same time, he started to work as a handyman for a dentist who had grown to like him(!!!), so he could pay for his dental reconstruction.

The change was confirmed to me one day while I was waiting for another patient in the waiting room of the Mental Hygiene Center. A nurse I worked with asked me, "What did you do to Daniel? I have known him for years and he is completely changed."

"Well, he's still quite a character," I answered awkwardly.

"Flavio, you don't understand. Daniel is a different person."

I started to realize that it was true. After a year and a half, I was facing an insolent and cheeky[6] man, but now an adult man. His jeans and T-shirt were not torn and mis-sized, his hair was combed, not a hint of bad smell, and his grin now more frequently opened into a smile. Above all, he had learned how to have healthier interactions, less arrogant and in-your-face, without any violence. The "pleasure" he felt in beating people and the danger of being sent back to prison were just distant memories.

After a while, Daniel decided to go back to Sicily. With his trademark pride and insolence, he said that he had nothing else to do in Rome. And so, he let on, he was going back home, to his mother, and that he would find a way to start again.

Notes

1 The title "A Violent Life" is a homage to *Una Vita Violenta*, a 1958 novel by the Italian writer/filmmaker Pier Paolo Pasolini, which was later made into a movie in Italian (1961) and French (2017).

2 This was also a variant of the classic solution-focused *observation task* (de Shazer, 1988; Hoyt & Berg, 1998, p. 331) designed to change the viewing of the problem, although in SFBT such tasks are typically directives to observe or notice something positive rather than to notice something risky or undesirable.

3 These logics are specific to Brief Therapy. With other approaches, like Cognitive Behavior Therapy or psychodynamic therapies, some techniques may fall under the logics I already identified (so that those logics would be *universal*, so to speak, or transtheoretical), whereas others would involve different kinds of logics. That is because different logics of intervention correspond to different epistemological theories. As Nardone and Watzlawick (2005, pp. 39–40) have written: "There is not only one reality but many realities, determined by the perspective of the observer and by the instruments used for observation.... For the clinician, theories must not be irrefutable truths, but hypotheses related to the world, partial points of view, useful for describing and organizing observable data so as to achieve successful therapies or to correct unsuccessful ones."

4 For an in-depth explanation of the idea of the attempted solution, see Watzlawick et al. (1974).

5 The definition of reframing offered by Watzlawick et al. (1974, p. 95): "To reframe, then, means to change the conceptual and/or emotional setting or viewpoint in relation to which a situation is experienced and to place it in another frame which fits the 'facts' of the same concrete situation equally well or even better, and thereby changes its entire meaning."

6 To use a British term. American English speakers might prefer "impudent or irreverent, typically in an endearing or amusing way."

References

Budman, S.H., Hoyt, M.F., & Friedman, S. (Eds.). *The first session in brief therapy*. New York: Guilford Press.

Cannistrá, F. (2018, December 6). *The nine logics beneath brief therapy interventions.* Short course, Brief Therapy Conference, Burlingame, CA: sponsored by Milton H. Erickson Foundation.

Cannistrá, F., & Piccirilli, F. (Eds.). (2018). *Single session therapy. Principles and practice*. Florence, Italy: Giunti. (Published in Italian as *La terapia a seduta singola. Principi e pratiche.*)

de Shazer, S. (1988). *Clues: Investigating solutions in brief therapy*. New York: Norton.

de Shazer, S., Dolan, Y.M., Korman, H., Trepper, R., MacCollum, E. & Berg, I.K. (2006). *More than miracles: The state of art of solution-focused therapy*. New York: Haworth.

Duncan, B.L., Miller, S.D., Wampold, B.E., & Hubble, M.A. (Eds.). (2010). *The heart and soul of change: Delivering what works in therapy* (2nd ed.). Washington, DC: APA Books.

Erickson, M.H. (1967). *Advanced techniques of hypnosis and therapy: Selected papers of Milton H. Erickson, M.D.* (J. Haley, Ed.). New York and London: Grune & Stratton.

Erickson, M.H. (1980). *Collected papers* (Vols. 1–4; E.L. Rossi, Ed.). New York: Irvington.

Fisch, R., Weakland, J.H. & Segal, L. (1982). *The tactics of change. Doing therapy briefly*. San Francisco: Jossey-Bass.

Green, D.J. (1995). Persuasive public speaking: How MRI changed the way I preach. In J.H. Weakland & W.A. Ray (Eds.), *Propagations: Thirty years of influence from the Mental Research Institute* (pp. 227–242). New York: Haworth Press.

Hoyt, M.F. (2009). *Brief psychotherapy: Principles and practices.* Phoenix, AZ: Zeig, Tucker, & Theisen. (Published in Italian as *Psicoterapie brevi. Principi e pratiche.* Rome: Centro Informazione Stampa Universitaria [CISU], 2018.)

Hoyt, M.F. (2017). *Brief therapy and beyond: Stories, language, love, hope, and time.* New York: Routledge.

Hoyt, M.F., & Berg, I.K. (1998). Solution-focused couple therapy: Helping clients construct self-fulfilling realities. In M.F. Hoyt (Ed.), *The handbook of constructive therapies: Innovative approaches from leading practitioners* (pp. 314–340). San Francisco: Jossey-Bass.

Nardone, G., & Watzlawick, P. (1993). *The art of change.* San Francisco: Jossey-Bass.

Nardone, G., & Watzlawick, P. (2005). *Brief strategic therapy: Philosophy, techniques, and research.* New York: Jason Aronson.

Norcross, J. C. (2010). The therapeutic relationship. In Duncan, B.L., Miller, S.D., Wampold, B. E. & Hubble, M.A. (Eds.), *The heart and soul of change* (2nd ed., pp. 113–142). Washington, DC: American Psychological Association.

O'Connell, B. (2012). *Solution-focused therapy.* New York: Sage.

Patrick, C.J. (2013). The therapeutic expression of anger: Emotionally expressive writing and exposure. *Theses and Dissertations, Paper 238.* University of Wisconsin-Milwaukee.

Pennebaker, J.W. (1997). Writing about emotional experiences as a therapeutic process. *Psychological Science, 8*(3), 162–166.

Pennebaker, J.W., & Beall, S.K. (1986). Confronting a traumatic event: Toward an understanding of inhibition and disease. *Journal of Abnormal Psychology, 95*(3), 274–281.

Shapiro, D. (1965). *Neurotic styles.* New York: Basic Books.

Short, D., Erickson, B.A., & Klein, R.E. (2005). *Hope and resiliency: Understanding the psychotherapeutic strategies of Milton H. Erickson, M.D.* Norwalk, CT: Crown House Publishing.

von Foerster, H. (1984). On co-constructing a reality. In P. Watzlawick (Ed.), *The invented reality* (pp. 41–62). New York: Norton.

Watzlawick, P. (1978). *The language of change: Elements of therapeutic communication.* New York: Norton.

Watzlawick, P. (Ed.). (1984). *The invented reality: How do we know what we believe we know (contributions to constructivism)?* New York: Norton.

Watzlawick, P., Beavin, J.H., & Jackson, D.D. (1967). *Pragmatics of human communication.* New York: Norton.

Watzlawick, P., Weakland, J.H., & Fisch, R. (1974). *Change: Principles of problem formation and problem resolution.* New York: Norton.

Weeks, G.R. (Ed.). (2012). *Promoting change through paradoxical therapy* (rev. ed.). Chevy Chase, MD: International Psychotherapy Institute.

Weeks, G.R., & L'Abate, L. (1982). *Paradoxical psychotherapy.* New York: Brunner/ Mazel.

CHAPTER **6**

Transforming Trauma and the Migration of Identity
Accepting the "Call" from Outside the Cave
Jim Duvall

Many current understandings about trauma make a direct link between trauma and psychological pain that can often lead therapists to incapacitating and pathologizing conclusions. "These understandings also lead to the construction of a fragile or vulnerable sense of self, and leave people with a keen sense that their person is ever susceptible to being trespassed upon in ways that they will be hard-pressed to defend themselves against" (White, 2005a, pp. 19–22).

In this chapter I will describe the chilling journey of a woman who experienced the debilitating effects of ritual abuse she suffered many years earlier. The unrelenting terror, psychological pain and emotional distress she was left with as an outcome of the trauma will be revealed. The pathologizing discourses of mental-health professionals and her husband dismissed the debilitating effects of her traumatic experiences, plunging her into the depths of a shadowy, ever-present, frozen story where she remained in the grips of isolation, fear, and despair. She spent many years stalled in her attempts to find any ways to move forward in her life, until one day, she was called upon to face the very fears, isolation, and despair that had taken over her life.

A collaborative therapeutic conversation, grounded in narrative practices and a rites-of-passage metaphor (Van Gennep, 1960; Turner, 1977; White, 2007; White & Epston, 1990; Duvall & Béres, 2011) was offered as an alternative way of engaging with her about the traumatic effects. Because of the "call," which is an element of a rites-of-passage metaphor, her story began to move forward toward a future of hope and possibility. Through this emotionally charged, high-stakes conversation, she was invited to get in touch with her hopes for the future and options for taking steps to move forward in her life. By facing her fears, it became possible for her to gain control of them, break free from the isolation of her internal "cave" and begin to more fully inhabit her life.

Act 1: Separation Phase and Responding to the "Call"

I had just returned to the Institute from a meeting at another agency when I was told that a woman who had appeared without an appointment was sitting in the waiting room asking to see me. The receptionist was concerned that she looked frightened and very fragile and that I should see her immediately. When I arrived in the waiting room I found Elaine sitting with her head down, hands clasped together and clutching a tattered piece of tissue. Her hair and clothes were a mess and clearly, she had been crying profusely. She was barely making eye contact with me and her voice was faint. She repeatedly whispered, *"I'm sorry, I'm wasting your time."* I knelt in front of her, looked up into her eyes and said, *"I'm glad you came. Why don't we go to my office?"*

I had met with Elaine, her husband and son for a few sessions some months prior. A school counsellor initially referred them because their nine-year-old son, Nathan, was experiencing anxiety and had expressed that he wanted to end his life. After meeting several times, he appeared calmer, more engaged with his peers at school, and refocused on his schoolwork.

We arrived at my office and Elaine took a seat in the corner of the room. Again, her head was down, and she barely made eye contact. Leaning forward in her chair and staring at the floor with her hands tightly clasped on her knees, she was breathing heavily and her right leg was vibrating. We sat together in silence for over 10 minutes. Finally, I asked:

Jim: Elaine, what needs to happen here for this time we have together to be useful?

Elaine: It's hard to breathe and to talk. I'm sorry. I shouldn't be here.

Jim: Take as much time as you need. [*hands her a bottle of water.*]

Elaine continued to stare at the floor for a long period of time. It struck me that she was unaware that she had become my unpaid supervisor. I was learning a lot from her about listening, patience, and the use of silence and recognizing her pain as a testimony to what she gave significant value to in her life (White, 2005a). For her to come to my office in this emotional state meant that there must have been something very important for her to talk about. I realized that I had to find a way to go as slow as possible, and then go even slower. She began to speak:

Elaine: I learned from watching Nathan, in our sessions with you, that he had picked up my ways of coping and being in the world. I realize now that he wanted to end his life because of being around me. He has a right to be healthy, happy and have a good life. I have to get better so that he can have a chance to be healthy and happy.

Jim: When you say, "so that he can have a chance to be healthy and happy," it gets me thinking about what that says about your ideas about what it means to be a mother? What values does that reflect that you want Nathan to be healthy and happy? Also, it gets me wondering, do you think you have a right to be healthy and happy, too?

Elaine: I've been like this for so long that it's become my life and who I am. I feel like I'm lost. Jim, I live in an ever-present, dark and bleak world.

Jim: Elaine, would it be useful if you told me what's going on? What happened?

Elaine: You're asking me to tell you what happened to me? That would be very tough and frightening to do. My own husband doesn't believe me.

Jim: Yes, of course, it would be tough to do. Elaine, it seems like you have an important story to tell. I want to understand it so that I can be useful to you. So, even though it would be tough and frightening to do, can you do it anyway?

Elaine: [*minutes pass as she stares straight ahead with her eyes welled up with tears*] I'll try, but I don't want you to judge me. I'm always worried that I will slip into the cave for the final time, never to return.

Jim: I only want to understand what's happened so that I can try to be useful to you.

Elaine: [*breathing heavily, her eyes continuing to tear up*] This is so hard to say to you. I'm so ashamed of what happened to me. Years ago, in the late 1980s I was ritually abused by a cult. I was physically and sexually abused repeatedly over a long period of time. It was painful, humiliating and ter-rifying. There were times I thought I was going to die. I was also forced to watch them abuse other children and animals. There were so many of them, men and women, and they wore robes and hoods so that I couldn't tell who they were. I lived in a farmhouse just outside of a small town and couldn't trust anyone in town because I couldn't identify the members in the cult. They could have been anyone in town.

Jim: Elaine, that sounds horrible. Given what you experienced, how did you even manage to cope with day-to-day life?

Elaine: I had a dog named Chief. Chief was a collie and he was my best friend. It didn't matter what emotional state I was in, he was always loving and affectionate toward me. I felt safe with Chief. When I was with him I could steal moments in time when I could escape from the sheer terror of the cult members. I learned to get away from them by fleeing into my inter-nal world. I called it my cave. I found refuge by retreating into the cave, and I still do, but it leaves me very isolated, lonely and disconnected from friends and family.

Jim: So, you felt safe with Chief and you learned to briefly escape from the ter-ror of the cult members by retreating to your internal world that you call the cave. And, although it provided temporary refuge it also left you iso-lated and unavailable to the connections and emotional support of your family and friends.

Elaine: Yes.

Jim: What other effects of the abuse remain with you today?

Elaine: I get flooded with memories and dark purple shadowy images of the cult members in their robes. They constantly float and swim around in my head. I try to escape them and retreat further into my cave. But, then I'm even more disconnected from others around me. My psychiatrist told me that I have Dissociative Identity Disorder [DID: see Lynn et al., 2012]. To this day I'm absolutely terrified of being around groups of people and avoid them at all cost.

Jim: So, you become flooded with dark purple shadowy images of the cult members in their robes and they constantly swim around in your head. It sounds like fear and terror take up a lot of space during those times. Sometimes they even push you further into the "cave." And to this day, you are frightened of groups and want to avoid groups at all cost. Do I understand you correctly?

Frequent paraphrasing and summarizing provided a reflecting surface, letting Elaine know that I got it. I intentionally used her words to reduce any distortion due to my interpretations. If I didn't understand her correctly, the summaries provided opportunities for her to correct and adjust me as we proceeded with our conversation.

Elaine: Yes. And, sometimes it's been so frequent and intense that I have thought of just ending it all and taking my life. I've even thought of how I would do it. I could finally have peace, and everyone would be better off without me.

Jim: You could kill yourself if you really wanted to. Elaine, how did you get this far? You're here today. What stopped you?

Elaine: My love for Nathan. That's what keeps me going.

Jim: So, what keeps you going is your love for Nathan.

Elaine: Yes, but I realized that I need help to get better. I'm constantly tormented. I desperately need to get a life. This is bigger than what I can do on my own. I need help to do this.

Jim: What ideas do you have about what "help" would look like?

Elaine: It was helpful when you met with us as a family. Nathan is calmer. He no longer talks about ending his life. He's reconnected with his friends again. He's interested in his schoolwork again. You know, it has been hard for me to trust anyone at all. But, after being with you in the family sessions, I was thinking maybe I could begin to learn how to trust again, with you. That's why I just came here today. I really want help. If I don't get help with overcoming these intense relentless fears I honestly don't know if I can make it.

Jim: Elaine, given what you have been through, it seems completely reasonable to me that you would have a hard time trusting anyone. However,
I want to make sure that I understand you so far. I would like to take a
minute to summarize ... members of an organized cult physically and
sexually abused you many years ago. You were humiliated and terror-
ized and at times even thought you might die. They also forced you to
witness the abuse of other children and animals. Many years later they
continue to take up space in your life as dark purple shadowy images
swimming around in your head. As a result of their continued presence you have fled into your internal "cave" more and more. It is there
that you find refuge from the relentless fear and terror and the unwieldy
presence of the dark purple shadowy images of the cult members. Yet,
even though the cave offers you refuge, it also isolates you from supportive connections with your family and friends. And, you have lived in this
isolated, reclusive existence for many years. From what you're telling me
the isolation has amplified, and you are even more disconnected from
the support of your family and friends. Finally, you said that to this day
you are terrified of groups and avoid them at all cost. Do I understand
you so far?

Elaine: Yes, that sums it up.

It was becoming clear to me that Elaine needed to face her fears and get
them in front her. If she were in relationship with her fears she could stand up
to them and manage them. For many years she had been left to endure her fears
in isolation. In a therapeutic context I could offer her the support and scaffolding required to embark on this journey toward the life she preferred. I could
recruit an outsider witnessing team that would both offer her support and help
to deconstruct the strong negative attributions she associated with groups of
people that were linked to her experience of being abused by the cult.

My concern was that Elaine was in a highly anxious and vulnerable state and
there was a risk that she would panic and reject the idea of therapy that included
an outsider witnessing team all together. In addition, I had a tentative level of
connection with her and we were likely to engage in an emotionally charged
dilemma. I did not want her to have a "knee-jerk" reaction out of fear and abandon the possibility of working with me. I also wondered about the ethics of
suggesting the involvement of a group and might it create risk for her. I finally
concluded that as her experience was intensifying, it would create more risk
for her and Nathan should she continue to retreat internally and become more
disconnected from family and friends. So, I decided to offer the "call" and tell her
clearly that I thought we needed to include a group in the therapeutic process.
Then I needed to be prepared for a strong reaction from her and to immediately
respond with support and understanding. Clearly, it was about to become an
emotionally charged, high-stakes conversation.

The "Call"

Jim: Elaine, I'm happy to see you for therapy. However, there is an additional aspect to the therapy process that I think is critical. That is that it's very important that a group joins us for the therapy sessions.

Elaine: [*Her eyes immediately widened, she leaned forward and had an alarmed look on her face.*] What? I can't believe you said that! You can't be serious. That's a horrific thing to say! I just told you that I'm terrified of groups and avoid them at all cost!

Jim: It's understandable that you are reacting this strongly after what you have been through. Elaine, what may have been a realistic initial response to your fears years ago no longer seems to be serving you well years later. I understand from you that your fears have become increasingly intense, more frequently present, unwieldy and taking up more space in your life. I'm concerned that your continued retreat from them is giving them more power over you. You have become increasingly more isolated and disconnected from family members and friends. My proposal to include a group in the therapy process must have come as a bit of a shock. However, one significant difference now is that this time you wouldn't be doing it alone. I would work alongside you and support you to corral your fears and get them in front of you so that you can address them. If you are in relationship with your fears you can increase your control over them rather than them controlling you.

Elaine, I'm offering you a way to practice being with a group. You can view it as practice for real life. The group would be a team who would sit behind a one-way mirror and listen to our conversation. At some point during the conversation we would switch places with them. They would go into the therapy room and we would go behind the one-way mirror where you can listen to what they have to say. They would not offer judgments. It is not an assessment. They would simply comment on what stood out for them in our conversation together. We call this a reflective practice. Many families who come for therapy here find it useful.

Elaine: It just seems horrifying! What if I get frightened and escape more into my cave?

Jim: Tell me if there is something I can do to help if that starts to happen. We can go as slow as is necessary and take one small step at a time.

Elaine: Well, it will be a first time ever that someone would be right there with me to support me. I still find it intimidating but just having you there would make a difference. If there is anything else you could do I'm sure it will come to me.

I offered Elaine the "call" (Campbell, 1968) and invited her to separate from an "aspect of her identity that is determined no longer viable" (White &

Epston, 1990, p. 7; White, 1999) and to embark on a quest. This call of involving a group in the therapeutic process would be 180 degrees from her history of avoiding her fears. This journey begins by separating from known and familiar beliefs and practices (Turner, 1977; van Gennep, 1960) and moves toward what is possible to know and do. This represents Act 1 of the metaphor of the 3-Act Play (Duvall & Béres, 2011), a rites-of-passage comparison. The metaphor of a 3-Act Play has been used previously as a framework for conceptualizing therapy. There are similarities between the use of the 3-Act Play in Resource Focused Therapy (RFT) (Ray & Keeney, 1993) and Narrative Therapy (White, 1990; Duvall & Béres, 2011). They also speak about movement away from problem states.

In RFT, the goal of Act 1 is to get out of it and move into the next one, Act 2. In most plays, the middle act is the transformational hinge, linking the beginning to the end. The final act, Act 3, is for plays with resourceful endings, a situation of resolution and generativity (Ray & Keeney, 1993, p. 3).

This use of the 3-Act Play metaphor in narrative practices is distinct in that it is intended to serve as an organizing concept for universal story form. *Story* is a central concept and the *raison d'être* of a narrative practices approach. "This universal story form spans generations across time and traverses many cultures" (Duvall & Béres, 2011, p. 27). The three sequenced stages form, known as the *rite of passage*, has a beginning, middle and ending. Act 1 is the separation (preliminal) stage in which the problem is understood within social and cultural context and the person is often presented with a "call" to embark on a journey. Act 2 is the journey (liminal) phase, which is wrought with ambiguity, challenges, and new learnings. Act 3 is the post-liminal stage, in which the person experiences a re-incorporation of identity, integrating values and skills from the pre-problem past with new learnings acquired through the journey phase. It is important to note that eliciting someone's story in order to bring forth coherence and meaning is not an anything-goes process. van Gennep proposed that the three sequenced phases contain both process and structure. Offering Elaine the "call" made it possible for her to think away from what she routinely thought and represented the beginning of an incremental scaffolding process to create movement forward.

Outsider Witnessing Practices

This reflective practice structures rituals that are acknowledging of and "regrading" of people's lives, in contrast to many of the common rituals of modern culture that are judging and degrading people's lives (White, 2005b, p. 15). Rather than retreating into her internal world and facing her fears in isolation with all of the demoralizing effects, Elaine could face her fears with the support of the outsider witnessing team and myself and experience the remoralizing effects. The shaping of her identity becomes a public and social achievement (White, 2005b; Meyerhoff, 1986). As Elaine's internal hopes, dreams and commitments are known in the external world they can be acknowledged, thereby increasing the possibility of their "stickability" (Duvall & Young, 2009). The outsider witnessing team would offer Elaine the experience of a group that would have the opposite effects of the group who ritually abused her. There would be a principle of transparency. The outsider witnessing team, through the process of telling and retelling, would notice and thicken the subordinate story lines that have been hidden in the shadows of Elaine's life. They would identify small acts of living (Wade, 1997) and initiatives that may have gone unnoticed and are then thickened into rich counter-plots and that contribute to a robust sense of identity. These are ways of validating Elaine's preferences for living, moving the subordinate story forward, and making visible new options for action that were not previously available.

These reflective practices and the development of the Reflecting Team originated through the work of Tom Anderson and his colleagues in Norway (Anderson, 1991). Later, Michael White, drawing from the work of cultural anthropologist Barbara Myerhoff (1980) and his own work with Aboriginal cultures in Australia, developed the practice of outsider witnessing teams. The outsider witnessing teams differ from Andersen's original version of the reflecting team with structure and categories of inquiry (White, 2000).

Act 2: The Journey Phase

We scheduled the next session. I arranged for an outsider witnessing team to join us. My colleagues at the Institute and I served as outsider witness team members during each other's sessions. In this way team members were consistent and dependable as we were all trained in that particular way of practicing and were familiar with each other.

Elaine had accepted the "call" and we tentatively began our journey toward what was possible for Elaine to know and do while breaking free from a life filled with fear and isolation. I asked Elaine if we could name her journey as a project. She named it the *"Getting My Life Back Project."*

Before we began the session, I asked Elaine to join me behind the one-way mirror to meet the team members. Before meeting her the team members were reminded to use only their first names and refrain from using credentials. They were encouraged to bring more of their personhood forward in order to be more visible to Elaine.

I introduced her in the following manner: "Hi everyone, I would like to introduce you to Elaine. We are inviting you to travel along with us on Elaine's journey to get her life back." Each team member shook her hand and greeted her with a comment to generate transparency and resonance such as "I'm also a parent "or "I have a nine-year-old son as well." Elaine smiled timidly and made tentative eye contact. When we entered the therapy room, I asked her:

Jim: Elaine, how are you doing so far?

Elaine: Right now, it feels a bit nerve-racking. But, they all seem like pleasant people.

Jim: These are your sessions; we can go at your speed.

They were asked to listen within four categories of inquiry (White, 2005b, p. 17) and be prepared to interview each other in the therapy room with Elaine listening to them behind the one-way mirror. This structure evolved from the poststructuralist idea that identity is a social and public achievement.

Elaine attended seven sessions with the outsider witnessing team and 12 sessions in total. The process was challenging, but not threatening. As the therapy progressed she became more confident in her abilities and more committed to her hopes and dreams. There were also many actions that she incrementally initiated in order to practice standing up to her fears during the Act 2, as follows:

She respectfully confronted a waiter who was rude to her and her friends.

- He apologized for his performance and invited her and her friends to return and promised friendly service in the future. Her friends said that they were impressed with the way she handled a difficult situation.
- She confronted her husband when he was emotionally abusive to their son. He responded by saying, "I don't care what you think, I'm his father and I can do whatever I want." She spoke with me about it in the following session and described how she just "froze" and didn't know what to do. I said, "Does getting your life back depend on people always agreeing with you?" The following week she addressed him again. She said, "You cannot continue treating our son in that emotionally abusive manner, period. It's not open for discussion." He followed by sending her a card and flowers. She said in the following session that she felt like she was coming out of her cave and beginning to get her life back.

These are two small examples of many trial and error initiatives that Elaine performed as practice to finally face her intense debilitating fears, which were the purple shadowy images swimming around in her internal world.

Act 3: The Re-Incorporation of Identity

Elaine arrived at the ninth session prepared to face her biggest fears, the purple shadowy images of her abusers. She said she was ready to get her fears in front of her and stand up to them.

Jim: What ideas do you have about how to get your fears in front of you?

Elaine: I'm going to close my eyes and allow their images to appear. Then, rather than retreating to the cave, I'll face them in protest and confidence. Having you in the room with me will help to give me strength.

Jim: Of course, just tell me how I can be useful.

Elaine closed her eyes and they remained closed for approximately five minutes when tears began streaming down her face and her right leg was vibrating. Her eyes remained closed for about ten minutes. As she slowly reopened her eyes she had a faint smile on her face. She said, "For years I've been frozen in the ever-present and now I feel like I can just throw doors open and run through them."

The next session, I asked:

Jim: Elaine, what values or skills lie in the past [pre-problem] that would be useful to bring forward and integrate with the new learning and skills that you have acquired on your journey to get your life back? What was it about you at that time that you appreciated about yourself and that others appreciated about you?

Elaine: (looking up and pausing) I was a very persistent person. I had real stick-to-it-ness. I liked the challenge of doing things that were a bit harder or a bit more complicated. I was also creative. I was an accomplished musician and even played in clubs. But I haven't touched my guitar for a very long time. It's been stored in the attic for many years.

Jim: If you brought persistence and creativity forward into your present life, would that be part of the project of getting your life back?

Elaine: Absolutely, yes! I'm getting excited as I think about it.

Jim: Could you give that some thought between now and the next time we see each other? Then we can discuss what ideas you have come up with.

Elaine: Yes. I'm looking forward to it.

Elaine returned two weeks later and was excited to talk about what had evolved in the preceding two weeks.

Jim: You look like you've got something to say. Why don't you start the conversation today?

Elaine: Well, after we talked I really got thinking about my guitar and how great I used to feel when I played it. As soon as I got home I went up to the attic and got it. I was so happy to see it. It was in rough shape from sitting up in the attic all those years. So, I took it to a music store where they are bringing the wood back and reworking the fret board. It's been so long since I have played I feel very rusty, so I have arranged lessons with a music teacher. I am so looking forward to playing music again.

Elaine also resurrected a journal that had been lying dormant since prior to her abuse. She began writing in it again and said that as she watched the words appear on the pages, it was like watching herself reappear in her life. Through perseverance and careful scaffolding, she was able to face her fears, escape from isolation and renew connections with her friends and family members.

Conclusion

This brief example offers an illustration of Act 1, Act 2, and Act 3 of the 3-Act Play (Duvall & Béres, 2007, 2011) rites of passage metaphor (Turner, 1977; van Gennep, 1960; White, 1990) as a structure and process to engage with Elaine, a woman who had suffered the debilitating effects from ritual abuse which occurred many years earlier. Her response to the "call," including her willingness to confront her fears in front of a group of witnesses, freed her to cross the threshold, progressively distancing her from a frozen story of fear and despair toward an alternative story accelerated by forward movement and hope for the future.

References

Anderson, T. (1991). *The reflecting team: Dialogues and dialogues about dialogues.* New York: Norton.

Campbell, J. (1968). *The hero with a thousand faces.* Princeton, NJ: Princeton University Press. (Original work published in 1949.)

Duvall, J., & Béres L. (2007). Movement of identities: A map for therapeutic conversations about trauma. In C. Brown & T. A Scott (Eds.) *Narrative therapy: Making meaning, making lives* (pp. 229-250) Thousand Oaks, CA: Sage.

Duvall, J., & Béres L. (2011). *Innovations in narrative therapy: Connecting practice, training and research.* New York: Norton.

Duvall, J., & Young, K., (2009). Keeping faith: A conversation with Michael White. *Journal of Systemic Therapies*, 28(1), 1–18.

Lynn, S.J., Berg, J., Lilienfeld S.O., Merckelbach, H., Giesbrecht, T, Accardi, M., & Cleere, C. (2012). Dissociative disorders. In M. Hersen &; D.C. Beidel (Eds.), *Adult psychopathology and diagnosis* (pp. 497–538). New York: Wiley.

Myerhoff, B. (1986). Life not death in Venice: Its second life. In V. Turner & E. Bruner (Eds). *The anthropology of experience* (pp. 261–289). Chicago: University of Illinois Press.

Myerhoff, B. (1980). *Number our days: Culture and community among elderly Jews in an American ghetto.* New York: Touchstone/ Simon & Shuster.

Ray, W., & Keeney, B. (1993). *Resource focused therapy.* London: Karnac Books

Turner, V. (1977). *The ritual process: Structure and anti-structure.* Ithaca, NY: Cornell University Press. (Original work published 1969.)

van Gennep, A. (1960). *The rites of passage.* Chicago. University of Chicago Press. (Original work published 1909.)

Wade, A. (1997). *Small acts of living: Everyday resistance to violence and other forms of oppression.* New York: Human Sciences Press.

White, M. (April, 1999). *Migration of identity map in narrative therapy.* Three-day training operated by Brief Therapy Training Centre-International (a division of Hincks-Dellcrest Centre, Gail Appel Institute), Toronto, Ontario, Canada.

White, M. (2000). *Reflections on narrative practices: Essays and interviews Adelaide,* Australia: Dulwich Centre Publications

White, M. (2005a). *Attending to the consequences of trauma.* (workshop notes) Adelaide, Australia: www.dulwichcentre.com.au.

White, M. (2005b) *Definitional ceremony and outsider witness responses.* (workshop notes) Adelaide, Australia: www.dulwichcentre.com.au.

White, M. (2007). *Maps of narrative practice.* New York: Norton.

White, M., & Epston, D. (1990). *Narrative means to therapeutic ends.* New York: Norton.

CHAPTER 7

Heating Up to Cool Down
An *En*countering Approach to Ericksonian Hypnotherapy and Brief Therapy

Douglas Flemons

Edgy and exhausted from continually failing to control his body's stress response, Azran – "Az" – was referred to me by a therapist who'd tried unsuccessfully to help him with hypnosis-infused relaxation training. Any time Az had to deal with someone he deemed an "authority figure" – a teacher, coach, supervisor, cop, doctor – he would become hyper-alert and self-conscious, which was soon followed by intense anxiety. The same sensitivity would arise whenever he felt another person's eyes staring at him. Unfortunately, this was not an infrequent occurrence, as he had the face of a movie star and the powerful build of a professional athlete. An accomplished tennis player and gifted graduate student, he moved gracefully and spoke eloquently.

Az's shift to a heightened, reflexive focus was triggered by either the social status or lingering scrutiny of others, but it was jet-fueled by his anticipation and dread of what people would think of him once they noticed what typically happened next. Beads of sweat would form on his forehead, and then, when he failed to calm his pounding heart or contain his mounting panic, his thoughts would race and his whole body would heat up. He could, he said, "soak through a shirt in two minutes flat." His previous therapist had offered hypnotic imagery of cool locations and breezes to counteract this automatic response. When he could picture such conditions during their sessions, it helped him feel more comfortable, he said, but it didn't make a difference outside the office.

Az and his family had immigrated to the US eight years earlier, when the political situation in his home country had become untenable. Eighteen months prior to their leaving, back when Az was 16, his older brother, driving alone, was detained at a military checkpoint. A search of his car was initiated. A scuffle ensued. A severe beating followed, and then imprisonment. Some months later, while still in custody, long before any trial, Az's brother died.

A few months after the funeral, Az was in a car with some friends when they were pulled over for speeding. As the policeman approached the driver-side window, Az, sitting in the backseat, started trembling. Somehow he managed not to draw the officer's attention, but by the time his friend had offered a sufficient bribe and they'd been waved back into traffic, Az felt spent and his clothes were drenched.

Now, nine years later, Az, living in the States, wasn't sure he could continue pursuing his graduate studies. He believed his current struggles traced back to what happened to his brother, but his symptoms involved more than the trembling and sweating he experienced that day in the backseat of his friend's car, and they could be set off by virtually anyone – authority figures, sure, but also family, friends, neighbors, fellow students, and both tennis opponents and tennis partners. The person didn't even have to be in his presence; he'd sometimes start having a panic attack and get tongue-tied while talking on the phone. He felt so impossibly caught and interpersonally shut down, he'd been thinking about suicide. His mother, recognizing his struggle and self-doubt, was afraid for him; his father was just disappointed and critical. He told Az that he needed to "get control" of himself.

The previous therapist's strategy of offering hypnosis-induced relaxation training was well meaning and no doubt skillfully delivered. But the logic informing the approach was in keeping with what Az had already been frantically doing on his own – trying to tamp down or counteract his symptoms. Relaxation necessarily involves a softening, a letting go. But when it is raised as a shield to protect against frantic, visceral sensations, or when it is thrust as a sword to smite unrelenting anxious thoughts, it freezes into something hard and brittle, rendering it useless—nothing more than an experiential oxymoron. So rather than signing on to help Az *counter* his thoughts and visceral symptoms, I committed to helping him *encounter* them instead. I didn't explain this, didn't say it directly; rather, my commitment was implicit in what I asked, described, invited, and suggested. The organizing principle of my engagement was what Milton Erickson (1980) called *utilization*. I approached Az's sweating, ricocheting thoughts, and fast-beating heart as *abilities* that, if effectively applied, refined, or tweaked could themselves serve as pathways to the amelioration of his suffering. Ericksonian hypnosis and the logic informing it are ideally suited for inviting such alterations.

Az and I met for three sessions, each 90 minutes long. Our time together was interlaced with hypnotic interactions, though I seldom labelled them as such. Az hadn't been demonstrably helped by his previous experience of hypnotherapy, so I wanted to mark what we were doing as somehow different. I thus offered no formal hypnotic inductions (e.g., "As I count backwards from ten to one, you can feel yourself moving deeper and deeper into trance"), and I never suggested that he close his eyes and relax. His finely tuned, non-volitional mind-body connection was very much in evidence in his hair-trigger visceral responses to challenging circumstances. It only made (Ericksonian) sense, then, to utilize these easily evoked reactions as efficient segues into mini therapeutic trances. Az could never quite put his finger on what was happening to his body as we worked together, and, as you'll see below, he was never quite comfortable with the process, but he could tell that something significant was shifting – something he was unable, but also didn't need, to control.

Early on in the first session, I told Az a story of an initiate who went to Nepal to study with a Buddhist teacher. The monk literally lived in a cave in the mountains, so he recognized the urgent necessity of his new student's learning to use meditation to raise his body temperature. The young man would need to master the skill in order to survive the fast-approaching winter. "Isn't it interesting?" I mused, "What you already know how to do automatically, the student had to travel all the way to Nepal to learn." He laughed nervously and said, "Let's go the other way. Let's cool me down."

Az's worried appeal for "going the other way" was predicated on the rational idea that problems are best dealt with by counteracting or avoiding them. However, a utilization approach is predicated on the *relational* idea that problems are best dealt with by *en*counteracting them – by approaching and engaging them. Typically, clients, and those who fail to help them, attempt to solve problems via negation (e.g., in this case, *preventing* or *stopping* heating up), substitution (e.g., *going in pursuit* of cooling down *as opposed to* heating up) or symmetrical battle (e.g., *pitting* cooling down *against* heating up). In contrast, utilization-informed therapists invite therapeutic change via acceptance (e.g., *allowing* heating up), inclusion (e.g., *embracing* both cooling down *and* heating up as legitimate), and complementary (circular) engagement (e.g., *arriving* at cooling down *by way of* heating up).

Over my three sessions with Az, I used anecdotes and experiments to invite shifts toward acceptance, inclusion, and circularity. The first experiment, designed for him to fail, helped him reconsider his, and his father's, assumption that what he needed was more control over his body.

Douglas: Would you like to do an experiment?

Azran: Okay.

Douglas: Okay, can you purposefully raise the temperature of your forehead right now? Not by imagining something, just by you consciously making it happen, by saying to your forehead, "Okay, temperature, up you go."

Azran: [After some time spent trying] No.

Douglas: Try harder. Use more willpower. Demand it.

Azran: [After several seconds] I can't do it.

Douglas: Gives you a sense of why that meditation student had to head to Nepal. Okay, can you purposefully speed up your heart?

Azran: [After several seconds] Can't do that either.

Douglas: No. You've been thinking something was wrong because you can't, on cue, cool your forehead or slow your pulse. But you can't heat or speed up your body, either. Not on purpose…You can't police your body.

Azran: As hard as I try.

Douglas: Right! Your body isn't going to let anyone mess with it – not your dad, not even you.

Rather than try to protect Az from his symptoms by helping him arm himself against them, I invited his panicky thoughts and body reactions into our sessions, both directly and indirectly, so he could practice relating to them differently – relating to them resourcefully rather than fearfully. Az dated the beginning of his problem to the time the police officer was walking toward the car he was riding in as a teenager, and of course this followed the death of his brother at the hands of the military. With this in mind, I evoked the presence of such authorities through my metaphoric language choices ("you can't police your body"), and I made sure to sip my tea out of a cup that had the initials *FBI* prominently displayed on the side. Near the end of the first session, I asked him, "So, is it okay for your conscious mind to take off the badge?" He said it was.

Paying attention to such contextual details is integral to relational sensitivity and a relational sensibility, one that accounts for and utilizes details of both the inter- and intra-personal relationships composing the client's experience. I heard in Az's voice the anger and frustration he felt in response to his father's dismissive belief that Az wasn't strong or determined enough to get his symptoms under control.

Azran: He thinks I should just buck up.

Douglas: He thinks if you only try harder, you'll be able to beat it.

Azran: Yes.

Douglas: Your body understands that bucking up, fighting back, doesn't help – it actually makes it worse.

Azran: My father doesn't.

Douglas: Your father doesn't understand that, no.

What better, more satisfying, way for a young man to come into his own, to find his confidence, his bearing, than in contradistinction to an overly critical father, a father that didn't, and probably could never, understand? What better way to launch into trusting, rather than fighting against, his body?

The naming of conditions of suffering – e.g., "anxiety," "panic attacks," "depression," and such – facilitates short-hand communication and understanding among clinicians, as well as between them and their clients or patients. On the surface, this seems sensible, nothing more than an efficient summing-up. But such naming concretizes classes of symptoms as stand-alone entities, prepackaged with a set of cultural and personal preconceptions and expectancies about the frustrating irrationality and intractability of them. Considered formidable, uncontrollable opponents, such entities – categories of mental illness – are therefore commonly assumed (by clients and clinicians alike) to require powerful counteracting interventions to wrestle them into submission. No wonder brain-altering, side-effect-inducing medications seem so alluring.

Implicit, and therefore invisible, in such characterizations is the assumption that the process of addressing mental-health problems entails doing something *to* them. I choose instead to do something *with* them. This is, after all, the essential therapeutic shift in orientation inherent in Ericksonian utilization. But I don't take the classified whole of the problem as a given. That is, I don't attempt to do something with such entities as "anxiety" or "panic attacks." Instead, I work with (more, *play* with) the contextualizing definitions of problems, as well as the non-volitional *composing strands of experience* that get clustered into such categories. I'm interested in the details, the blood-and-guts descriptions of visceral, tangible, identifiable thoughts, actions, sensations, feelings, emotions, and images. I am thus curious about instances of, for example, pain, temper, despair, fainting, desire, urges, disgust, crying, flashbacks, sweating, nightmares, cramping, nausea, dizziness, temperature shifts, heart-quickening, humiliation, hyperventilating, perseverating thoughts, and/or hallucinated voices and images. It is important to underscore that none of these experiential strands can themselves be considered as stand-alone "things"; they are all noted and articulated in the interactive, self-fulfilling swirl of expectation, perception, interpretation, and response that recursively defines intrapersonal communication, conscious awareness, and interpersonal conversation. This is why they are all amenable to change, to therapeutic alteration – they aren't isolable *entities*, they are *patterns* of intra- and interpersonal interaction. Introduce a difference somewhere in the unfolding of such patterns, and it, and the difference it makes, can ramify. That's how therapeutic change typically happens – it starts small and extends out of the office and into a life.

Having experientially discovered that he couldn't purposefully lower *or raise* his temperature or heart rate, Az was amenable to experimenting with a different approach.

Douglas: Like other elite athletes, you have a highly refined mind-body connection. When you're on the tennis court, your conscious mind doesn't issue orders to your feet and your shoulders and your arms and your grip. You rely on a virtually instantaneous, integrated coordination between different parts of your body – right hand and left foot, left eye and right hand, right hip and left shoulder – and between all of these parts and your awareness. When you're in the zone, it's all effortless.

Azran: Yes. Very much.

Douglas: Being in the zone, being in sync with your mind-body coordination, is an excellent way to learn. Hypnosis is just a means for getting in the zone without having to be on a tennis court.

Azran: Okay.

Anecdotes and stories allow ideas to be offered and considered analogically, rather than analytically. The fabric of them, the pattern organizing them, implicitly communicates a shift in orientation, a shift in relationship between the person and his or her experience (Flemons, 2002). The following story and the experiments that evolved out of it illustrate the process:

Douglas: I once directed a clinic that developed an air-conditioning problem. Actually, the AC in most of the building was just fine. But the largest room, the one where we met for staff meetings and group supervision, it got to where it was way too cold all the time. Anyone who was going to be in there for any length of time made sure to bring a sweater; otherwise, it was unbearable. Over the course of a year, we probably had the AC guy come out half a dozen times, and every time he told us the same thing in the same irritated, authoritative voice: "Nothing is broken: the condenser checks out, the air handler is fine, and the thermostat isn't stuck." But my staff and I were still miserable, so I asked the office manager to call yet again. I guess the usual guy was away, or maybe he was sick of dealing with us. Anyway, a new technician comes out, and he does the usual equipment check, and then he does something the other guy didn't. He comes and stands with me in the cold room. Doesn't say anything, just stands there, feeling the temperature, looking around the room. And then he asks, "How long has that floor lamp been there in the corner, next to the thermostat?" I think for a while. "Oh, I don't know, I guess about the same amount of time that we've been freezing our asses off."

Azran: [laughs and continues looking at me]

Douglas: The heat from the lamp was perpetually warming the air right next to the thermostat, so from the thermostat's perspective, the room was never cold enough to trigger it to send a signal turning off the AC. Once we moved the lamp, the AC would cool down the room *and* the thermostat, and when that lower-level threshold on the thermostat was reached, it tripped a switch and the AC would turn off, just like it was supposed to. This would allow the room to start warming up, and when the thermostat registered that the roomed had warmed sufficiently, when the upper-level threshold had been reached, it sent a signal that fired up the AC, and the room started cooling down again. Just like it was designed to do. The room had to cool down enough for the thermostat to know it was time for it to begin warming up, and it had to warm up to the necessary threshold before the thermostat could send the signal to start the cooling process. For the thermostat, it's all just a circle: you cool down *so* you can heat up, and you heat up *so* you can cool down. Let's facilitate your body remembering, or learning perhaps for the first time in a long time, how to heat up till you reach that threshold where your metabolism, your internal thermostat, triggers an automatic cooling down. Instead of trying to make it happen, you can just allow your body to activate the balance of that circular process.

Azran: Okay.

Douglas: So you can just become aware of my eyes looking at you.

This was my invitation to Az to go into trance; nothing more was needed.

Azran: [nervously laughs] Oh, I just knew you were going to do something twisted.

Douglas: [laughs] Is that okay? Are you okay registering the fact that I, in my twisted way, am looking at you?

Notice my use of the word "registering," which I'd used when talking about the thermostat.

Azran: Yeah, it's okay.

Douglas: You're comfortable with feeling uncomfortable?

Azran: [laughs] Yeah, well, no, but okay.

Douglas: Great, so as you notice my eyes, even focusing on them, what else are you registering?

Azran: My heart is beating faster.

Douglas: Yes! Excellent! What else?

Azran: I'm heating up…

Douglas: Yes, your heart and your temperature can work together that way. Faster and hotter, hand in hand, heart and head, faster and hotter.

Azran: I can feel your eyes on me. That's what's killing me.

Douglas: Good.

Azran: Oh boy, *[laughing]* this is rough. Ahhh.

Douglas: What's happening?

Azran: Oh, it's still going.

Douglas: Oh, it is.

Azran: Yeah, 'cause I can feel like your eyes on it and I can't stop it.

Douglas: Terrific, so go ahead and look at me.

Azran: [laughs] I don't want to look at you.

Douglas: I know you don't.

Azran: [laughs]

Douglas: Just allow it to continue until the upper-level threshold is reached and your internal thermostat sends the signal to automatically initiate the cooling and the slowing process. Keep heating up till you reach that threshold. I don't know if the signal will first be from your heart, registering that it got fast enough to trigger the slowing down... Or whether your heart will get the message second-hand from your forehead, or from somewhere else in your body, that the upper-temperature threshold has been reached and the cooling down process has been triggered. In which case the slowing of the heart can be fast on the heels of the cooling down.

Azran: That's crazy.

Douglas: What's crazy?

Azran: I got cool.

Douglas: Cool. So, what happened?

Azran: I felt your eyes on me, and I just started heating up.

Douglas: Terrific. And what happened then?

Azran: I don't know, I just relaxed.

Douglas: Ah-ha.

Azran: I don't know. I can't explain it.

Douglas: You can't explain it consciously, but your body understands it.

Azran: It's happening again right now, but it's not as bad.

Douglas: Great. Keep looking at me, then. Allow your body to recycle this learning again and again. With more practice, it just becomes second nature. Just like in tennis. It's one thing to understand this intellectually. Now you've shifted to knowing it in your body, viscerally. You've shifted to unconsciously employing it. A kind of tennis knowing. I don't know if your conscious mind will ever figure out what your body already knows.

Azran: Oh, it just happened again.

In that first 90-minute session, Az later said he had a "double-digit number of panic attacks," that is, times when his heart and his temperature rocketed up. And each time, he'd reach an upper-limit threshold that triggered a slowing of his heart and a cooling of his body. It got so that by the end of the appointment, the cooling would start before he broke a sweat. He left gratified but also troubled. In the second session, he explained why.

Azran: I really didn't want to come here. But this is helping.

Douglas: Talk to me about the not wanting to come.

Azran: I still don't understand it, but the attacks are so fast from hot to cold, it's awesome.

Douglas: Yeah...

Azran: But double-edged.

Douglas: What is double-edged about it?

Azran: I don't understand why it starts in the first place.

Douglas: And if you understood it?

Azran: I'd stop it.

Az hated not knowing why he heated up, and he hated not understanding how his body was able to automatically cool down. We devoted much of the session to running more hypnotic experiments so that at least his body could "get the hang of it."

During the third and last appointment, we had the following conversation:

Azran: I don't know what you did to me *[laughs],* but it's good.

Douglas: Well, I don't know that I did anything *to* you. I think your body has figured out a different way of getting comfortable.

Azran: I'm amazed. But I'm not cured.

Douglas: What does that mean?

Azran: I'll still feel the heat. But it goes away. So. And the fact that I have no voluntary control of stopping. I hate that.

I reiterated my view that striving for voluntary control isn't necessary or helpful.

Azran: [laughs] Yeah.

Douglas: Last time you found it disconcerting that you couldn't understand how it was happening. So, can you be comfortable going into the future, saying "that was some weird shit [we did]?"

Azran: [laughs!] Yes, I can, I can.

Douglas: All right. You're an academic, so of course you want an intellectual understanding. But you can forgo that?

Azran: Yes.

Douglas: You're sure? You can be comfortable with your body figuring it out?

Azran: Yes, because it happens so fast. It's amazing.

Douglas: Sounds like your body has discovered the wisdom of circles.

Az described his mother as "elated" at the changes she had seen. She was "glowing" at seeing his life back on track. His father, predictably, was not effusive. But Az could meet the gaze of other people, his words weren't getting tangled when talking to his professors or classmates, and his body reliably knew how to heat up to cool down.

Six months after our last appointment, I was leaving a store, walking to my car, when I heard someone calling my name. I turned and saw Azran, waving and then striding across the parking lot towards me. We shook hands. Smiling, he said, "I guess you can tell by how dry my grip is how well I'm doing."

Clinical theorists sometimes construe successful counterintuitive interventions as paradoxical, postulating that there is something inherently helpful or healing about "paradoxing" clients (e.g., Selvini-Palazzoli, Boscolo, Cechin, & Prata, 1978; Watzlawick, Weakland, & Fisch, 1974). I take a different view. To my mind, the stories and experiments in this case were *en*counterintuitive – that is, they fit a way of approaching therapeutic change that privileges acceptance and inclusion of, and complementary engagement with, clients and the idiosyncratic patterns of their problematic experiences. What transpired only appears paradoxical if viewed from the outside perspective of conventional rationality. From the inside perspective of therapeutic *relation*ality, my client and I extemporaneously and collaboratively explored and discovered what can happen when symptoms are embraced as vehicles for, rather than shunned as roadblocks to, resolution and change.

References

Erickson, M. H. (1980). Further clinical techniques of hypnosis: Utilization techniques. In E. L. Rossi (Ed.), *The collected papers of Milton H. Erickson: Vol. 1* (pp. 177–205). New York: Irvington.

Flemons, D. (2002). *Of one mind: The logic of hypnosis, the practice of therapy.* New York: Norton.

Selvini-Palazzoli, M., Boscolo, L., Cecchin, G., & Prata, G. (1978). *Paradox and counter-paradox.* New York: Aronson.

Watzlawick, P., Weakland, J., & Fisch, R. (1974). *Change: Principles of problem formation and problem resolution.* New York: Norton.

CHAPTER 8

Looking "Outside the Box" for Client Strengths[1]

Joseph A. Goldfield

Early in my career I studied strategic family therapy, receiving advanced training with Jay Haley (1977, 1980) and Cloé Madanes (1981,1984). They, of course, were influenced by the psychiatrist Milton Erickson (1980; also see Goldfield, 1994; Haley, 1973, 1985), who advocated that clinicians accept and "utilize" their patients' symptoms; I went on to study Ericksonian approaches with Jeff Zeig and Stephen Gilligan (see Goldfield, 1994, 2003). I also absorbed ideas from the Mental Research Institute (MRI: Watzlawick, Weakland, & Fisch, 1974; Fisch, Weakland, & Segal, 1982) about positive feedback loops, unsuccessful attempted solutions, and second-order change; as well as concepts from Salvador Minuchin (1976; Minuchin, Rosman, & Baker, 1978) about hierarchies and family structure. Later, I was also influenced by the competence-emphasizing ideas of solution-focused brief therapy (SFBT: de Shazer, 1985, 1988; Berg, 1994) and the re-storying concepts of narrative therapy (White & Epston, 1990; see Goldfield, 1993, 1998a, 1998b, 2013; Ronch & Goldfield, 2003).

With each case I try to integrate these ideas in ways that will help the particular client. In challenging and potentially high-risk situations, when there may be the temptation to hunker down, is often just when we need especially to think creatively.[2] At such times it helps me to recall what Stephen Gilligan, elegantly paraphrasing Erickson,[3] told me long ago (personal communication, 1991): "Not knowing [what to do] is the calling card of the unconscious."

Here are three examples that involve "outside the box" interventions.

Example #1: Following the Smoke – and Not Getting Mesmerized by the Flames

In 1988 I was the new social worker for six adolescent boys living at a residential treatment center in Northern California. I had been at the group home for three weeks. On the third Monday, I got a call that one of the boys, Tommy, age 13, had set a fire at school. The fire was in a small trashcan and was extinguished quickly without injury or damage. I was told that Tommy had a background of setting fires. The staff and administrators were extremely concerned about this behavior. Indeed, one of the primary goals written into Tommy's formal record by his state caseworker was to reduce this behavior and to have Tommy develop safer ways of dealing with stress. This behavior also was one of the factors preventing Tommy, who had been at the group home for about a year, from being considered for family reunification.

In my first two weeks I had been getting acquainted with the boys in my office as well as observing them together at the group home. Tommy appeared serious and a bit distracted. Smaller than the other boys, he nonetheless was respected by them. His roommate, the oldest and most powerful, was protective of Tommy and kept an eye out for him

Tommy's teacher informed me that Tommy had dyslexia and some learning disabilities, as well as other expressive language deficits, and was receiving special education services for these problems.

At the time of this particular fire, no one could identify what might have triggered the incident. Coincidentally, I was scheduled to see Tommy that day for his regularly scheduled session. In light of the recent fire incident, I needed to give this serious thought.

I recalled how Cloé Madanes (1981, pp. 84–85) had a mother teach her firesetting son how to light a fire and put it out correctly, and that she had used that as a daily activity for the mother and son to spend time with each other. I thought of the strategic therapy idea that behavioral problems of youth often reflect an inverted hierarchy in the normal family structure wherein the youth has power over the parents rather than the other way around. Although we weren't dealing with an inverted family hierarchy, it seemed that the situation had some parallels in that those in authority were unable to control Tommy's fire setting and he was able to control them. Although it was a different context, I extrapolated that some version of what Cloé had done might work to restore the hierarchy at the group home by my assuming the parental-teacher role myself.

With these principles in mind, I prepared for Tommy's session. By the time he arrived, I had set up a bowl of water on top of a metal card table and put this safely in the center of the room. I had also placed a pad of paper and some matches on the table. Upon his arrival I asked Tommy if he wanted to play a game I thought he would have fun with. He said "Yes," so I ushered him to the bowl of water, handed him the matches, and asked him if he knew "at least one really cool way to light a match and put it out safely?" He said that he did, and I asked him would he show me? He lit a match and put it into the water

I acknowledged that that was a cool way. I then tore a piece of paper from the pad, firmly rolled it up, and asked if he knew at least one way to light up that piece of paper and put it out safely? He said that he did and proceeded to demonstrate. Again, I acknowledged his skill. Then I tore a second piece of paper from the pad and asked him if he could tell me all the people and places he would like to see on fire? I offered to help by writing them down on the paper. He gave me a list. I wrote it down and double-checked that it was complete. Then I said, "You know, Tommy, it's kind of like these people and places are now on this paper." He agreed to this idea. I then firmly rolled up that piece of paper with the list and asked if he knew at least one way to light it up and put it out safely – which he did. After acknowledging his skill, I asked if he liked that game, to which he replied, "It was really cool." We made a deal that if I did not hear of any other incidents of fire-setting during the week we could play it again in the following session.

We then went back to the area in my office where I would usually sit and have sessions. Tommy spoke at length about wanting to see his mother. He hadn't seen her in a long time. She lived at the other end of the state and didn't have the means to come and stay for a weekend in order for them to have a family visit. I told him that I would look into it and see if there was anything I could possibly do to expedite a visit.

At the session the following week, I had the table and bowl of water placed again in a safe part of the office. I told Tommy that I hadn't heard of any incidents of fire-setting during the week, so we could play the game again. He asked if it was OK if we didn't, and could I take him to the video arcade instead? I got clearance from my supervisor. On the way, he asked if we could get some pizza. We did, as it seemed a more natural and comfortable environment in which to hang out and get to know each other. I discovered that Tommy loved playing the game "Pacman" but was only rarely able to go and play because living in the group home prevented having access to the game. He told me he might be rusty as he hadn't played it in a while.

Once at the arcade, I discovered that Tommy did not have any cognitive deficits with Pacman. He was highly skilled and demonstrated enormous eye-hand coordination, dexterity, and speed. He seemed absorbed and to be fully enjoying himself as he continued to advance to new levels of difficulty. As I watched, I thought about the idea of hierarchy and how a 13-year-old asking for and receiving permission to have pizza and to be taken to a video arcade was a much better way for him to navigate stressors than setting fires and rattling adults.

For the following two years many of our sessions involved going for pizza and to the video arcade. During those sessions I would often discuss various stressors in my life and the ways I navigated them, successfully or not. Although Tommy was not verbally expressive, he could still learn peripherally and indirectly. On occasions when we saw kids or other people having conflicts, we would discuss ways to handle conflict situations. For a few months I would always have the table with bowl of water and matches set up in the safe part of the office and would ask Tommy occasionally if he wanted to play that game. He usually declined, enough so that after a while I didn't set up the rigging but told him if he ever wanted or needed to, we could play it.

I also was fortunate enough to be able to facilitate bringing Tommy's mother up to the area a few times a year. We were able to cover the costs of transportation and a hotel so that Tommy was able to have weekend visits with her. Tommy had been removed permanently from her home and was now a ward of the state, and during my phone interactions with her it became clear she was very unlikely to be able to learn the skills needed to set limits in a way Tommy could respond positively to, so I kept the focus of our discussion on having good interactions and her expressing support regarding Tommy's desired behaviors.

Comment. When I presented this case to the other social workers at the residential facility, I was asked why I had not handled the case in a more traditional way, e.g., initially teaching Tommy a vocabulary for his feelings and then how verbally to express these feelings in a safe way? One reason was because teaching him a new way to think and express himself would be a long-term process in the best of circumstances and I wanted to intervene quickly due to the risks of the fire-setting. A "let's learn to talk about feelings" approach had not worked thus far, and I didn't want to repeat unsuccessful attempts (MRI) or do more of what doesn't work (SFBT). I knew that he was more an action-oriented than a verbal person. Since he was drawn to fire, I wanted to find a safe way to engage with him around that. I thought that if I could acknowledge his skills with his primary coping mechanisms, over time he might be more receptive to other gradual, longer-term skill development. I felt I would not be sensitive to who he was if I started off by trying to get him to master very complicated and subtle verbal skills on top of the basic age-appropriate ones with which he was already struggling. I also felt that at age 13, he could use an adult male role model (similar to a Big Brother) who was interested in him and was consistently available and supportive. The pizza parlor and video arcade provided a nice setting for me to verbalize and present him with various stressful situations and reasonable ways to handle them. This indirection would allow for what M.C. Bateson (1994) has called "learning along the way."

After that third week and until I left the job two years later, Tommy had no more fire-setting incidents. However, the day after I left that job I heard that he lit a match on the school bus and blew it out safely.

Example #2: Is There an Expert in the House?

Somewhat later, around 1990, I was working as a family therapist in the outpatient psychiatry department of a large hospital in a Midwestern city. One of the clinic's child and adolescent psychiatrists asked me to provide family therapy to the family of one of her patients.

Her patient, Jennifer, was a 13-year-old girl who was being treated for anorexia. She had been in the inpatient unit for two weeks and medically stabilized, then discharged to outpatient treatment. She had been in the outpatient program for about a month but was not making tangible progress.

The treatment team had initially included the psychiatrist and Jennifer's counselor, who provided individual and group therapy, as well as a nutritionist. Now, I was being added.

For a few months I met with the family on a weekly basis – both parents, Jennifer, and her older brother, a high-school student. The father, Richard, was a truck driver who frequently had to make hauls that kept him away from home for days at a time. The mother, Mary, was a stay-at-home mom and appeared to have become overwhelmed managing two adolescents, often alone without her husband's presence and support. Both parents and the brother, Bobby, described having urged Jennifer to eat more food and more healthily. They had tried placating her, accommodating to her shrinking list of acceptable foods. The parents had resorted to punishing her by restricting time with friends and telephone time, and also had used pleading and cajoling, but all to no avail. Jennifer was very good at school in terms of grades but didn't have many friends.

After a few months of the family therapy and other outpatient treatment, Jennifer was still not making significant progress – there was only most modest weight gain, she continued in maintaining strict control of what and how much she would eat, and there also was no discernable change in her extensive exercise routine of running and calisthenics. The family sessions also seemed stuck; the family focus was characterized by the parents and brother being helpless to do anything and fearing doing the wrong thing. The parents looked to me as an authority who would somehow influence Jennifer's behavior. I noticed that I was becoming inducted into that role, thinking of possible ways to directly change her behavior. I realized that I needed to go back to the drawing board

Jennifer really had the upper hand in terms of controlling her own eating behavior and of rendering the family helpless. I had no reason to think this was based on some hostility on her part, no evidence of abuse or extreme parental discord or punitive parenting. They were rendered passively helpless, like deer in the headlights. I therefore went with the assumption that it was a dynamic of an ongoing and mounting vicious positive feedback cycle of attempted solution by family and professionals and push-back assertion of independence by Jennifer. There was no solution to this Identified Patient taking on the world.

But, I thought, what if a second identified patient were introduced?

I surveyed the territory. I noted that her father, Richard, was considerably obese. While it might be conceived that her anorexia was a symbolic protest regarding his obesity, I did not know, but I thought that in any case I might be able to alter the impasse of family versus Jennifer in their battle over eating by switching our focus. They had gotten stuck and it seemed that a shock or jolt to the system was needed. I had learned from my teachers Haley and Madanes that when a child has assumed a parental role in a family, it is often better to make that hierarchy explicit. Perhaps it could be utilized?[4]

Wanting to see if the parents would cooperate and wanting to avoid a possible battle with them in front of their daughter, I called them in and discussed my plan that at the next family meeting I would berate the father regarding his obesity and his lifestyle choices that maintained this. He was desperate, so he gave me his permission.

At the next family session, the family began with the usual updates. I said, "Yeah, we can skip that for now. I have a different concern." I then turned toward the father and thoroughly lambasted him for not thinking of his family. I pointed out that he was overweight and clearly could be at cardiac and diabetic risk. He was sitting in the cab of a truck all day probably only stretching his legs at the truck stop where he certainly couldn't be eating wholesome food. What if he had a heart attack or stroke in his rig and lost control, subjecting himself and others to a dangerous freeway pile up?

Jennifer's father was slightly cowed as he let me scold him. He squeezed into his little chair, admitting I was right. He was ashamed for letting his family down. Jennifer looked shocked, her mother and brother remained silent. I quickly looked gravely at everybody, one at a time, and then stated, "Well, it seems to me that there is only one person in this room who is an expert on taking off the pounds and keeping them off."

I looked right at Jennifer. I told her that I knew she knew a lot about exercise but that she was still learning the basics of proper nutrition from her nutritionist. She said "Yes," so I said, *"OK, then can I put you in charge of your father's weight loss program?"* She agreed.

We went over some tasks that she would need to take on in monitoring her father's exercise and diet regimens. As we were finishing up the session, I told her, "Making these changes can be very hard for people, so don't be too rigid. But on the other hand, make sure he is adhering to the plan without giving him too many outs." (I had recognized an opportunity to give an indirect communication and suggestion to Jennifer about her own rigidity about her eating patterns.) This also allowed me to take myself out of a position of being in the middle of the power struggle and indeed to become a colleague on her side.

In ensuing family meetings, I continued focusing on the father's well-being and Jennifer's supervision of her father. If occasional dietary questions arose that neither she nor I had the answer to, I would refer her to her nutritionist. I had some further meetings with the parents and gave them praise and encouragement for how they were developing more effective ways of being protective and caring for their daughter.

I soon heard from Jennifer's psychiatrist and therapist that Jennifer began making more progress in her own treatment goals. Her weight gain was on track and she was becoming more engaged in her therapy group (often making helpful suggestions to other girls). She began spending more time doing adolescent activities with peers and became interested in age-related things like meeting a friend at the mall, discussing clique politics and boys, who were the mean versus nice teachers, etc.

Jennifer's father simultaneously began losing weight and exercising more. He announced that at his latest physical his primary-care physician had been impressed and encouraging. At the family sessions I heard more and more that some normalcy was returning to family life. Seeing Jennifer healthier helped the parents to become less frightened and frozen. The brother, who had dutifully attended every session, began coming less frequently; his parents said his attention was shifting from concern for his sister to making plans for college and seeing his friends more.

After a while, the parents felt that the family therapy was becoming less necessary, so we terminated it. Jennifer stayed in her group, however, which included a focus on relapse prevention, for another six months.

I heard from her mother a year later that Jennifer was doing well. She had made the freshman varsity basketball team. I was delighted that Jennifer was able to continue doing something she liked (exercise) for positive purposes, functioning as a member of a group, and using her competitive skills for a healthy activity. I was pleased that helping this family overcome their impasse allowed Jennifer to redirect her tendencies of control and being protective of her body and emerging personality to being protective of her family's well-being. She could be acknowledged as a maturing family member who was making a positive contribution while simultaneously dealing with the normal stressors of adolescence.

Example #3: Anger Management for Dummies

For many years, I have had a private practice in New York City. I frequently provide assessment and referrals and short-term counseling to clients through Employee Assistance Programs (EAPs) sponsored by their employers. Most are self-referrals for a wide range of issues. Occasionally they are work-mandated referrals based on performance issues or interpersonal work problems that need assessment and possible mental-health support.

Once I received a referral from the EAP of a large, well-known New York law firm. The manager's referral was for a long-term employee, Samuel, who worked in the firm's mailroom. Reportedly, Samuel had had recently gotten into a few verbal altercations with other employees, although generally he kept to himself and was serious about being good at his job. I was able to meet Samuel the following day.

Samuel was a 33-year-old man whose appearance was a bit striking. He was a tall, muscular African American man with thick, long, slightly unkempt dreadlocks. He wore army camouflage-style khakis, a wrinkled dress shirt, and a tie that seemed a bit small. He also wore extremely thick eyeglasses that made his eyes appear small and out of proportion to his face. He lived alone with his mother, who had chronic back issues and diabetes. He helped support her. He needed to keep his job, if possible.

Our initial conversation involved relatively standard assessment questions, including his understanding of why his company wanted him to speak with me. He told me that there were a few staff members, including one young lawyer, who had been disrespectful to him when he brought them their mail. He described people not thanking him, making irritated impatient statements, and being nonverbally disrespectful as they gestured condescendingly where to put the mail. He reported that he confronted them by either asking if they "had a problem," or by telling them they had better not disrespect him, or by sometimes telling them "not to act fucking condescending to me." Two occasions had resulted in voices being raised, leading to Human Resources issuing him a verbal warning and referring him to me.

When I asked if things ever got "physical," he said, "not at work." I asked what he meant, and he told me that he had gotten into a few physical altercations on the steps coming out of the subway. He recounted following someone who had pushed against him or looked disrespectfully at him and then hitting them and occasionally kicking and stomping them when they were down on the ground. He had avoided any legal consequences from these episodes as he knew how to melt into the rush-hour crowd.

I perceived Samuel to be a man who was under a lot of stress, caretaking his mother and being responsible for her and their economic well-being without his having many formal job skills. I also thought that he struggled with self-esteem issues, and that vulnerable self-esteem probably led him quickly to misperceive interactional events as a show of disrespect.

I explained that my job was primarily to "have his back" (meaning: look out for him). Following the solution-focused therapy approach with mandated clients (Berg & Miller, 1992), I asked what the job probably needed to see to know that his anger issues were resolved. We discussed what that would look like. Samuel said, "They'd have to see that I'm working on not getting into arguments." I asked if it would help if they knew he was in an anger management program.

He agreed, so I told him that I knew of a very respected anger management program in New York City. I really talked up the program – its excellent reputation and that I personally had a good, close relationship with the program director. I wanted to portray that joining that program would be a classy act. Samuel showed interest. I then asked if we could call them then and there to see if his insurance was accepted and also to see if they had immediate openings. I told Samuel that he would be able to hear exactly what was said, and when I asked if there was anything we had discussed that he would not want me to mention, he said I should tell my colleague everything.

We called and found out that his insurance was accepted, it was a 12-week program, and that he probably qualified but needed to have an intake with the director. He got that intake appointment scheduled for two days later, but unfortunately the next opening in the group wouldn't be for two weeks.

My sense was that he could handle the work situation okay for two weeks. I was really concerned about the subway/street situation, however, where people (including him) could be at serious risk. What to do?

I realized I had a copy of *Anger Management for Dummies* (Elliott & Smith, 2015) there in my office. I asked what he thought of maybe reading a standard book on anger management to start getting acquainted with some basic ideas and tools he would probably be learning in the program. He said he thought it would be a good idea. I asked that he not take offense by the "Dummies" in the title and said that they use the word on every book in the series. I said that I'd benefitted from the Dummies books on stress management, astronomy, and biology, and mentioned that when I first saw *Astronomy for Dummies,* I was turned off by the word "dummy" but eventually found the Dummies books interesting and well written for the layman and not in some condescending, pop-psych style. He was okay with giving *Anger Management for Dummies* a chance, so I handed him the book and asked if he wanted to peruse it for a few minutes.

As he read the book, Samuel held it straight up close against his face (possibly due to nearsightedness). I suddenly had a vision of him reading the book on the subway: a big rough-looking guy reading a book called *Anger Management for Dummies*! I imagined that the nonverbal message to not stare at or jostle this guy would be sent to any subway commuters, that this guy was really beginning to try to work on something and distracting him probably would not be a good idea.

I asked Samuel if he wanted to borrow it and said that he could return it after the other program started. I specifically suggested that he read it when on the subway, to distract himself from any possibly disrespectful people. I also said that reading the book could serve as an accessible toolbox for him in case some issue did arise on the subway.

Comment. The book and program would provide good information and support. The immediate target of my intervention, however, was the possibility of Samuel, who was already stressed and tense, mistaking an innocent look (due to self-esteem issues or perhaps eyesight problems, or both) on the subway as an insult and his being triggered and going on the attack. My strategy was that his holding up a book with the words "Anger Management" on the cover would encourage people to give him wide enough berth to reduce the chances of an interaction leading to a bad confrontation.

He returned the book, unscathed, when I saw him three weeks later. Samuel told me that he had read it frequently on the subway. He liked the anger management program leader and peers and said that lots of their ideas were really "deep." He also found that many of the program materials were similar to ideas in the book.

With Samuel's informed consent, I got periodic updates from the referral source. Samuel was doing much better. He was handling situations more calmly at work, enough to be able to stay employed. He successfully completed the 12-week anger management program. After receiving a certificate of graduation from that program, he continued intermittent involvement with the program. I believe that in this case, by not presenting myself as an expert and placing Samuel squarely in the driver's seat, I gave him the respect that he identified was so important to him, which made it easier for him to comply with what he needed to do to address his situation.

Conclusion

In each of the preceding cases, "out of the box" interventions helped Tommy, Jennifer, and Samuel to use their respective skills in ways that were healthier and brought them and those around them more peace and happiness. As I wrote in "Rapnotic Induction No. 1," the song in honor of John Weakland (Goldfield, 1993/1996, p. 371):

> It ain't that complex: problem resolution
> When you address the attempted solution
> When you do that change will happen fast
> There'll be no need to analyze what happened in the past.

Notes

1 The excerpts from "Rapnotic Induction No. 1" (Goldfield, 1993/1996) are © J.A. Goldfield 1993. Used by permission.

2 Before returning to school to get a MSW degree and become a psychiatric social worker, I worked in theater, including practicing mime and improvisation. One time I was on the subway in New York, and got off at the wrong station. I thought I could take a short-cut and walk to where I was trying to go, but a gang of thugs surrounded me and it looked very ominous – they were real nasty bad guys. One of them demanded my money. I was frightened and scared. I gave a quick fight-or-flight look around and saw that I could not flee, and certainly could not fight. I also realized that I wouldn't be able to talk my way out of this. Then I had a flash: Maybe I could mime my way out! I started pantomiming and acting like I physically could not speak. "Hey, he's a dummy [mute]" one of the gangbangers said sympathetically. I nodded, pointed at my mouth, and then gestured back and forth like I was lost and confused and didn't know where to go. I made some hand movements that looked like American Sign Language. The guys took pity – "Hey, we gotta help him, otherwise he's gonna get hurt [by another bunch of thugs]." They circled around me and walked me back to where I could get on the train and stayed to make sure I was safe until I was aboard and the train went down the tracks. It was quite a *You Said What?* moment – I surprised myself!

3 For example, Erickson (in Erickson & Lustig [1975] said: "It's important for you to realize that your unconscious mind can start a train of thought, and develop it without your conscious knowledge – and reach conclusions, and let your conscious mind become aware of those conclusions"; Erickson, Rossi, and Rossi (1976, p. 247) wrote: "We all have so much knowledge of which we are unaware" and (p. 155) "In the development of the human being learning in the unconscious became available in any time of need"; Erickson and Rossi (1979, p. 367) wrote: "Consciousness does

not have available all the knowledge that is in the unconscious" and (p. 203) "Your unconscious can know the answer, but you don't have to know the answer."

4 As I later said in "Rapnotic Induction No. 1," the song Insoo Berg had commissioned me to write and perform in honor of strategic therapist John Weakland at a conference held for him in New Orleans: "Make overt what before was tacit/Have 'em utilize their symptom as an asset!" (Goldfield, 1993/1996, p. 370).

References

Bateson, M.C. (1994). *Peripheral visions: Learning along the way*. New York: HarperCollins.

Berg, I.K., & Miller, S.D. (1992). *Working with the problem drinker: A solution focused approach*. New York: Norton.

de Shazer, S. (1985). *Keys to solution in brief therapy*. New York: Norton.

de Shazer, S. (1988). *Clues: Investigating solutions in brief therapy*. New York: Norton.

Elliott, C.H., & Smith, L.L. (2015). *Anger management for dummies* (2nd ed.). Hoboken, NJ: Wiley.

Erickson, M.H. (1980). *Collected papers* (Vols. 1–4; E.L. Rossi, Ed.). New York: Irvington.

Erickson, M.H., & Lustig, H. (1985). *The artistry of Milton H. Erickson*, M. D. Video/DVD. Bals Cynwyd, PA: Swan Media.

Erickson, M.H., & Rossi, E.L. (1979). *Hypnotherapy: An exploratory casebook*. New York: Irvington.

Erickson, M.H., Rossi, E.L., & Rossi, S.I. (1976). *Hypnotic realities: The induction of clinical hypnosis and forms of indirect suggestion*. New York: Irvington.

Fisch, R., Weakland, J.H., & Segal, L. (1982). *The tactics of change: Doing therapy briefly*. San Francisco: Jossey-Bass.

Goldfield, J.A. (1993). "Rapnotic Induction No. 1." *Journal of Systemic Therapies*, *12*(2), 89–91. Reprinted in M.F. Hoyt (Ed.), *Constructive therapies* (Vol. 2, pp. 370–371). New York: Guilford Press, 1996.

Goldfield, J.A. (1994, December). *A utilization approach for working with adolescents and their families*. Workshop held at the Sixth International Congress on Ericksonian Approaches to Hypnosis and Psychotherapy, Los Angeles.

Goldfield, J.A. (1998a). "The Master of Faster." In M.F. Hoyt (Ed.), *The handbook of constructive therapies* (pp. 243–245). San Francisco: Jossey-Bass.

Goldfield, J.A. (1998b). "The Problem Talks Back." In M.F. Hoyt (Ed.), *The handbook of constructive therapies* (pp. 245–248). San Francisco: Jossey-Bass.

Goldfield, J.A. (2003). Fundamental concepts of Milton H. Erickson and their relevance to older adults. In J.L. Ronch & J.A. Goldfield (Eds.). (2003). *Mental wellness in aging: Strengths-based approaches* (pp. 181–200). Baltimore, MD: Health Professions Press.

Goldfield, J.A. (2013). Off the couch and outside the box. In M.F. Hoyt (Ed.), *Therapist stories of inspiration, passion, and renewal: What's love got to do with it?* (pp. 87–99). New York: Routledge.

Haley, J. (1973). *Uncommon therapy: The psychiatric techniques of Milton H. Erickson, M.D.* New York: Norton.

Haley, J. (1977). *Problem-solving therapy: New strategies for effective family therapy*. San Francisco: Jossey-Bass.

Haley, J. (1980). *Leaving home: The therapy of disturbed young people.* New York: Brunner/Mazel.

Haley, J. (1985). *Conversations with Milton H. Erickson, M.D.* (Vols. 1–3). New York: Triangle Press.

Madanes, C. (1981). *Strategic family therapy.* San Francisco: Jossey-Bass.

Madanes, C. (1984). *Behind the one-way mirror.* San Francisco: Jossey-Bass.

Minuchin, S. (1976). *Families and family therapy.* Cambridge, MA: Harvard University Press.

Minuchin, S., Rosman, B.L., & Baker, L. (1978). *Psychosomatic families: Anorexia nervosa in context.* Cambridge, MA: Harvard University Press.

Ronch, J.L., & Goldfield, J.A. (Eds.) (2003). *Mental wellness in aging: Strengths-based approaches.* Baltimore, MD: Health Professions Press.

Watzlawick, P., Weakland, J.H., & Fisch, R. (1974). *Change: Principles of problem formation and problem resolution.* New York: Norton.

White, M., & Epston, D. (1990). *Narrative means to therapeutic ends.* New York: Norton.

CHAPTER 9

The Rock-n-Rollers Remixed

Back to the Future

Shelley Green

In 1988, Monte Bobele and I published a case study in the (then) *Journal of Strategic and Systemic Therapies*, entitled "An Interactional Approach to Marital Infidelity: Including the Other Woman in Therapy" (Green & Bobele, 1988).[1] The article described a less-than-conventional approach to couple's work when infidelity is the presenting issue, and the clinical work was grounded firmly in the foundational assumptions of the Mental Research Institute (MRI). At the time, I was a beginning family therapy doctoral student and Monte was my mentor. I was most fortunate to learn from Monte; I have always viewed him as the most MRI-ish person I've ever met – clinically and interpersonally. With his laid-back, one-down, three-moves-ahead therapeutic sensibility, Monte lives, breathes, and dances MRI principles and practices. And this case was a classic lesson for me in the elegant minimalism of interrupting solution attempts while honoring our clients' worldview (Watzlawick, Weakland, & Fisch, 1974).

This chapter first re-describes how Monte, the team, and I handled the case 30 years ago. The case was seen within the context of a university-based Family Therapy Clinic, where Monte supervised a team of six doctoral students behind the one-way mirror. Since that time, I have been teaching master's and doctoral students about systemic, brief therapies, and I've been co-developing brief therapy approaches to sex therapy (e.g., Green & Flemons, 2007, 2018; Flemons & Green, 2017, 2014). I've also spent the past 10 years developing a brief therapy-informed approach to equine-assisted psychotherapy (e.g., Green, 2013, 2014, 2017, 2018; Green, Rolleston, & Schroeder, 2018; Green, Schroeder, Rolleston, Penalva, & Judd, 2018). These projects have given me a perspective from which to re-examine what we did with this case and to imagine what I might do today if the same clients were to call me for a session.

The 1988 article is still a part of my assigned readings for the systems theories classes that I teach, and I refer to it frequently when teaching Human Sexuality and Gender. While I don't consider myself a pure MRI therapist, my clinical work is still significantly informed by the ideas that guided this case, and I find the assumptions congruent with so much of what still makes brief therapies unique, compelling, and effective. Here, I revisit that case with an eye towards the postmodern, social-constructionist, and relational ideas that guide my current work (Flemons & Green, 2014; Green, 2011, 2014; Green & Flemons, 2018), and explore how I might have intervened with this couple today.

The Original Case

This case was seen within the clinic that served as the training ground for doctoral students in Family Therapy in the late 1980s at Texas Tech University. Living in West Texas, where the values tended to be embedded fairly deeply in Bible Belt understandings, we often saw clients who expressed conservative views of marriage, family, sex, and commitment. It was a bit surprising, then, to meet our clients, Rick and Rhonda. Married for 14 years and with two children, they came to us concerned about Rick's ongoing, open affair with a woman who was 15 years his junior – the drummer in his rock and roll band. Rhonda had known of the affair from the beginning (over seven months when they presented for therapy), and had not challenged it until recently, when her nerves and her health had begun to suffer from the ongoing stress of dealing with Rick's attachment to another woman. The rationale for her long-term acceptance (or at least tolerance) of this affair was yet more surprising to our team; she and Rick not only described a totally open and honest relationship with each other – they also had a spiritual understanding of the nature of both their relationship and of the affair. As they explained it, they believed in reincarnation and knew that they had been together in several previous lifetimes. They also believed that Rick and his lover, J.J., had shared previous lifetimes and had in fact been twins in two earlier lives.

While I was fascinated by this couple's explanation of their beliefs in reincarnation and the pre-ordained, spiritual nature of their relationships – both with each other and between Rick and his lover – I returned behind the mirror at the break to find that my team was having a bit of trouble accepting this framework. Our team was comprised primarily of men (I had four male and one female doctoral student colleagues). At the break, several team members expressed their indignation that this man – a 34-year-old welder and musician – was not only wanting to "have his cake and eat it, too" but was actually succeeding. Some of my colleagues wanted to confront him on this, whereas others just wanted to complain at the unfairness of the situation. None of them initially believed his "cover" about reincarnation, but they were perhaps begrudgingly impressed that it was helping him justify maintaining two simultaneous relationships. I was concerned about Rhonda's emotional and physical health, as she was clearly suffering (she had lost over 70 pounds in the past seven months and was currently the family's sole source of income, as Rick had virtually stopped working), but I was also invested in exploring further her decision to let the affair run its course and allow Rick to decide in his own time.

Fortunately for us and for our clients, Monte was committed to the MRI principles of respecting the clients' worldview and of finding a way to interrupt the solution attempts that were maintaining the problem (Watzlawick et al., 1974). Behind the mirror, he invited us all to explore how Rhonda's commitment to the couple's belief in the timeless and inevitable nature of these intersecting relationships, as well as her desire to preserve the open and honest relationship she valued with Rick, prevented her from confronting Rick or demanding that he end the affair. In order to honor their deep love for each other, she refrained from pressuring Rick and was accommodating of his desire for frequent contact with J.J. As she told us, she assumed he would eventually come to his senses and return to their monogamous marital relationship.

We also explored, as a team,[2] the rationale behind Rick's solution attempts. He, too, was devoted to honoring the pre-ordained nature of both relationships and stated that his deep love for both women prevented him from choosing one over the other. As he explained, to choose one would devastate the other, and that was a choice he could not make. He saw no end to the dilemma, recognizing the distress it was creating, but believed that both women would wait for him indefinitely. Thus, our team came to understand how the solutions of all three involved perpetuated the couple's stuckness – the more Rick expressed his deep love for both Rhonda and J.J., the more devoted each woman became to expressing her reciprocal love for him by allowing him unlimited time to make his decision. We also came to understand how essential it would be for us to convey to the couple our complete respect for their unusual worldview, and thus for the unique nature of their relationships.

During the third session, Rick explained the exhausting and cyclical nature of the emotional reactions each of them experienced:

Rick: The emotions in this thing are incredible, because if you're getting what you want, then you can start feeling compassion for the other person. If you don't get what you want, you start feeling resentment for the same person because they're not giving it to you. And it just goes back and forth.

Shelley: And both of you are in those opposite roles at opposite times. One of you is resenting and the other is starting to feel compassion.

Rick: That seems to be the way it's working out.

In the same session, Rick shared further evidence of the other-worldly nature of their connection:

Rick: Ah!! Did you know that she (Rhonda) feels it when J.J. and I have sex?

Shelley: No.

Rick (to Rhonda): They never knew that.

Shelley (to Rhonda): Have you always? Physically?

Rhonda: Um-hmm.

Rick: To the second.

Shelley: So, you know when they are together and having sex, whether you would know it otherwise or not.

Rhonda: Yes, I was even in [another state] and I knew it.

Rick: She feels it.

Rhonda: By profusely sweating.

Shelley: How could you not be hung up on it when they are having sex far away and you're aware of it?

Rhonda: Uh-hmm.

Rick: But you try having sex with someone knowing somebody else is feeling it!

Rhonda: It's also something that I think after 14 years of marriage, something that should be shared with me.

This exchange intensified the team's understanding of the powerful connections these three experienced and enhanced our commitment to developing a path for therapy that would reflect our respect for their extraordinary, though painful, bonds. We were invested in avoiding "more of the same" solutions (Bobele, 1987) and in intervening in ways that could disrupt their continued oscillations. In the initial session, the idea of including J.J. in therapy had been briefly discussed but was met with reluctance from Rhonda (as well as from me – I could not imagine handling such intensity at that point in my clinical training). However, as we seemed to be as stuck as our clients, the team determined that a significant change was needed, and thus, the notion of including J.J. was again proposed as a way to interrupt the solution behaviors of both clients and therapist.

At our fourth session, with the team's encouragement, I tentatively introduced the idea of inviting J.J. to join a session. Rick was immediately on board, but Rhonda expressed reluctance and concern that this would take away from the focus on their marriage.

Shelley: The team observes that we've got two of the people in this intense relationship that involves three people …

Rick: Um-hmmm. I'd mentioned that early on that I'd like to see J.J. come in.

Shelley: Um-hmmm, they feel like we're going to be treading water and never getting anywhere until we have the whole relationship in here that we're dealing with.

Rhonda: I'm not real fond of that idea.

Rick: Why? That takes away some of our intimacy?

Rhonda: It takes away from (the idea) that she's not part of our marriage.

Rick: She's certainly having a large effect on it.

Shelley: Well, I see what you're saying, in that this is sort of sacred in here, because you're in here for marital therapy. And I can understand that. That is your bond here. If we were seeing just an ordinary married couple, the typical married couple with a mistress on the side, then we would never suggest that the husband bring his mistress in. Obviously, what you've got is an incredible bond here between the three of you. It's not the typical kind of situation. You two have a bond that is timeless and has gone on for lifetimes. And it's not the typical kind of marriage. So typically, we would not suggest this at all, but ...

Rick: So, it's an extraordinary case then.

Shelley: Well, it is, and I think we knew that from the time you came in that we're working with something really different here. And for that reason, we feel like if we don't have all three people involved, it will be difficult to get anywhere.

Rick: That's pretty well up to Rhonda.

Rhonda: What's the purpose of her coming?

Shelley: We've got someone that we're talking *about*, week after week, and we don't ever have her input, and obviously the two of you have really different sides to this relationship, different views of how this affects you. And I'm sure J.J. has her own view of how it affects her.

Rick: Right ...

Shelley: And we're not getting that information at all.

As this discussion continued, I offered a caveat to them about protecting their bond in such a session:

Shelley: But I think it would be very important for you both to feel comfortable to know that if we're going beyond your boundaries, that you would let us know.

Rhonda: Oh, I would.

Rick: Yeah, she's good about that.

In order to agree to including J.J., Rick and Rhonda had to be confident that we understood fully the unusual nature of their relationship and their struggle; this was pivotal, as others with whom they had discussed their dilemma had been dismissive, skeptical, and even openly mocking of their beliefs. The additional message of protection regarding their boundaries allowed Rhonda and Rick to affirm their ability and commitment to this and for Rhonda to feel a bit safer in agreeing to the joint session. This discussion with the couple exemplifies the two unique "You said *what*?" aspects of this case – our team demonstrated radical acceptance of the couple's unique belief system, and we chose to invite the "other woman" into the therapy setting. Both of these clinical decisions pushed the comfort zones of therapist, team, and clients, and both were primary elements in the progression of the case.

As the fifth and final session unfolded, I kept the focus of the conversation on the marital relationship and expressed the team's appreciation to J.J. for coming in to help us in working with Rick and Rhonda. Rhonda expressed a quite different stance immediately, appearing hostile and announcing that she had made her decision and was ready to ask Rick to leave the house. This significant difference in Rhonda's position represented the beginnings of change, and the team responded by doubting her ability to fully embrace change so dramatically so quickly. While Rhonda's stance had changed, Rick had become even more entrenched in his position that he was unable to decide between the women he loved. He shared openly his ultimate desire that both women could simply understand that he loved them both and wished to maintain both relationships.

Rick: It's not difficult for me to love either one of them. It's difficult for me to have them realize that I'm not loving them as much as they want.

Shelley: So it's hard for them to see ...

Rick: It's hard for me to deal with that. That's what keeps me in distress. I see J.J., and Rhonda gets upset. I see Rhonda, and J.J. gets upset. She doesn't show it as much, but it still bothers her.

Shelley: Okay, so correct me if I'm wrong ... Would the ideal situation be for both of them to just understand that you love both of them, and you could still have both relationships?

Rick: Yeah, that's what I've been doing.

Throughout this discussion, J.J. quietly expressed full support and patience for Rick as he took the time he needed to make a decision. When pressed by the team as to how much support she was willing to offer, she initially questioned whether we meant financial support (a level she seemed less willing to offer). However, she clarified that she would not pressure him to decide.

As the session closed, the team had a final message for Rick: they asked me to convey to him that they finally understood what he had been attempting to tell us – that he was in fact not capable of deciding between two women who he loved so much. I shared that we could see that the pressure we had all been applying on him to make a decision was in fact making things even worse for him.

Shelley: What we see is that you are in love with both women. At this point, you can't make a decision. You don't want to hurt either one of them and you don't want to give up either one of them. It's been going on for a very long time. You haven't been able to make a decision, and you can't make one right now. You cannot choose between them.

Rick: Um-hmm.

Shelley: But at the same time, it's pretty clear that this situation as it is right now can't go on forever. I know that for you, Rick, you can see that you would like to share both of them. If that would work for them, it would work for you. For right now, it's not working for any of you. But you can't make a decision. Since Rick can't make a decision, the two of you (*to the women*) are going to have to …

Rhonda: Um-hmm.

Shelley: So, what will happen, since Rick can't make a decision is that you'll decide …

Rhonda: Um-hmm, and I have.

Shelley: And you'll implement your decision.

We ended the session with Rick questioning how the women would be able to make a decision when he couldn't, but with Rhonda expressing firm conviction that she would have no trouble. This was a complete reversal for Rhonda, and our team believed it represented a second-order change in the ongoing solution attempts. It was, without a doubt, an uncomfortable end to a session for a beginning therapist. No one left the session happy.

Rick and Rhonda missed the next two scheduled sessions, and follow-up phone calls revealed that several changes had taken place, indicating their stalemate was coming to an end. In conversation with Rhonda, I learned that she was pursuing a job in another city, that Rick was currently living with J.J., and that she had informed him that if he decided his marriage and family were more important to him than J.J., he could come and join her. I offered her another appointment, which she declined. It was clear that her altered solution attempts were impacting all involved. I followed up with Rhonda again after a month, and she let me know of additional developments that pointed towards a reunification with Rick, without the continued involvement of J.J. While Rhonda had not moved cities for the job, Rick had experienced a series of difficulties, including a brief time in jail, that had, as Rhonda described, "made him think about how he was living his life." He had subsequently expressed his desire to end his relationship with J.J. and return to Rhonda and his family.

Rhonda's understanding of these significant changes resonated with the couple's unique worldview – she saw that Rick's recent "bad karma opened his eyes to the fact that one cannot live their life with total disregard for the lives of others." As she noted, Rick was currently attempting to help J.J. understand this, and Rhonda expressed her full confidence that she and Rick would be able to rebuild their strong and committed relationship.

The Rock-n-Rollers Today

It's a rare case that stays present in a clinician's mind for 30 years; this one has, and over the years Monte and I have affectionately referred to this couple as "the Rock-n-Rollers" as we have discussed the more compelling aspects of our work with them. We have both shown video of the case in our classes and invited our students to consider our choice of intervention. In my case, my students almost universally declare that they would *never* be willing to include the other woman in a couple's session. Some question the ethics of our decision, some wonder at our willingness to avoid challenging the couple's unusual belief system, and some simply believe inviting a lover into session would be "too hot to handle." I continue to be grateful for having had the opportunity to take risks, to explore the utility of fully embracing a client's unconventional worldview without judgment, and to attempt a second-order intervention.

As I review the case, I find some of my conversations and delivery to be awkward and unsophisticated (perhaps appropriate to my level of training at the time) and some of our language to be a bit quaint (e.g., *mistress!*). However, I continue to respect the commitment to honoring what our clients bring us, regardless of how it may differ from our own beliefs and ideas about relationships. And I am a bit in awe of our willingness at the time to utilize the clients' worldview to build an intervention that left them in significant discomfort.

One of the hallmarks of team-based interventions back then, influenced by the ideas and practices of the Milan Associates (Selvini Palazzoli, Cecchin, Prata, & Boscolo, 1978), was to deliver a message and quickly leave the room before the clients had an opportunity to deconstruct it. While I would not embrace this method now, I believe that our intervention conveyed respect for the clients' ability to choose their own path. Our investment was in change – but not in a specific direction that we either determined or advised. We attended to process rather than outcome. There is freedom in this stance for both the therapist and the client.

If this couple were to come to me for therapy now, I hope that I would be able to maintain my focus on process in order to avoid becoming invested in any specific outcome. I would still be interested in attending to attempted solutions – whenever I feel stuck with a case, this notion provides an anchor for me and helps me consider where and how to intervene. Such a focus is grounded in a non-normative, non-pathologizing stance that I believe is also consistent with the original case formulation. However, I would be more proactive in exploring the couple's dilemma from a strengths-based perspective. It would be important for me to highlight the systemic wisdom of the attempted solutions, and to punctuate the unique strengths that each of them brought to this long-term distressing situation. In this regard, my goal would be to continually make sense of their behaviors in context and to assume that they were each doing the only thing they could imagine doing, given the circumstances.

I can imagine asking how each of them had managed to maintain closeness with and respect for the other, given the intensity of the emotions involved. My conversations with them would be guided by genuine curiosity about how they imagined this situation playing out over time, and I would be less informed by a need to "intervene" and more attuned to how respectfully making sense of their behaviors could lead to increased relational freedom (Flemons, 2002; Flemons & Green, 2014, 2018) for each of them. My goal would be to alter their relationship to the problem, and I would assume that some transformation of their meanings and assumptions could take place in our conversation that would allow for second-order change – a change in the way they defined their relationship (Fraser & Solovey, 2018; Green, 2014).

If I were to envision a theme that might guide a useful second or third session with Rick and Rhonda – once I had established an understanding of and conveyed my respect for their beliefs about their relationships – it might be centered around the notion of integrity, and the conversation might unfold like this:

Shelley: It seems to me that you have each demonstrated a phenomenal ability to hold onto your own integrity in a very distressing and emotionally expensive situation. Rhonda, while you have clearly suffered tremendously over the past months, your commitment to Rick has not wavered, nor has your belief in the spiritual connection you share with him.

Rhonda: I know he loves me and I know we are meant to be together. No one promised it would always be easy.

Shelley: And Rick, as much as it hurts you to witness Rhonda's suffering, you maintain your belief in these two powerful relationships, and your trust in the integrity of your bond with Rhonda to withstand this emotional strain.

Rick: I have loved Rhonda in ways that I can never explain to anyone; I hate to see her in pain, but I love J.J. too and I can't pretend I don't.

Shelley: Yes, I see that. So, I wonder at the ways you will each find to continue holding onto your personal integrity while exploring the possibilities that these powerful relationships hold for you. It makes sense to me that Rhonda would not ask you to leave J.J. She understands the power of destiny and knows that you and J.J. have been brought together as well, regardless of how painful this may be for her. So, you both have an opportunity now to explore the potential of this integrity to guide you – to figure out how the presence of J.J. in your lives allows you to suffer, to grow, and to make decisions that honor all of you. It's quite powerful to witness your level of tolerance for suffering, and your belief that this will ultimately resolve in a way that fits for you.

Would I consider inviting J.J. into the session? Possibly, but not simply as a way to interrupt all of our solution attempts (including my own). If she did join us for a session, I might ask questions that addressed each of their belief systems and the implications and meanings attached to these beliefs. These questions might look something like this:

- What is it like for each of you, knowing that you have known each other in previous lives?
- What does this mean for your relationships now?
- Are specific patterns or decisions pre-destined?
- What is the role of personal autonomy or choice?
- Do your past lives and relationships, and the lessons learned there, have any bearing on the decisions you will make in this current incarnation?
- Do you imagine your paths will cross again in future lives? If so, what might this current dilemma mean for those new relationships?

I would be less invested in an intentional effort to alter their solution attempts, and more confident in my belief that honoring their current efforts could provide new opportunities for unique transformations – transformations that I could not predict but would certainly respect. Such commitments to discovery and respect were certainly at the forefront of Monte's teaching, and I hope that I have, in turn, passed them on to my own students. I suppose this is its own form of reincarnation – a generational renewal of the soul of effective therapy.

Notes

1 Some of the material contained herein originally appeared in S. Green and M. Bobele (1988), An interactional approach to marital infidelity: Including the other woman in therapy. *Journal of Strategic and Systemic Therapies, 7*(4), 35–47. Copyright © 1988 Guilford Press. Reprinted with permission of The Guilford Press.
2 The team consisted of Joe Strano, David Todtman, Rhonda Johnson, Paul Douthit, and Ron Chenail.

References

Bobele, M. (1987). Therapeutic interventions in life threatening situations. *Journal of Marriage and Family Therapy, 13*, 225–239.

Flemons, D. (2002). *Of one mind: The logic of hypnosis, the practice of therapy.* New York: Norton.

Flemons, D., & Green, S. (2014). Quickies: Single-session sex therapy. In M. F. Hoyt and M. Talmon (Eds.). *Capturing the moment: Single session therapy and walk-in services* (pp. 407–423). Bethel, CT: Crown House Publishing.

Flemons, D., & Green, S. (2017). Brief relational couple therapy. In J. L. Lebow, A. L. Chambers, & D. C. Breunlin (Eds.). *Encyclopedia of couple and family therapy.* New York: Springer. Retrieved from https://doi.org/10.1007/978-3-319-15877-8

Fraser, S. & Solovey, A. (2018). The process of change in brief sex therapy. In S. Green & D. Flemons (Eds.). *Quickies: The handbook of brief sex therapy* (3rd ed., pp. 70–98. New York: Norton.

Green, S. (2011). Power or pattern? A brief, relational approach. *Family Therapy Magazine*, *10*(6), 9–11.

Green, S. (2013). Horses and families: Bringing equine assisted approaches to family therapy. In A. Rambo, T. Boy, A. Schooley, & C. West (Eds.). *Family therapy review: Contrasting contemporary models* (pp. 256–258). New York: Routledge.

Green, S. (2014). Horse sense: Equine assisted single session consultations. In M.F. Hoyt and M. Talmon (Eds.). *Capturing the moment: Single session therapy and walk-in services* (pp. 425–440). Bethel, CT: Crown House Publishing.

Green, S. (2017). Equine assisted psychotherapy. In J. Carlson & S. Dermer (Eds.). *The SAGE encyclopedia of marriage, family, and couples counseling* (pp. 552–554). Thousand Oaks, CA: Sage.

Green, S. (2018). Partnering with horses to train mental health professionals. In K.S. Trotter & J. Baggerly (Eds.). *Equine assisted therapy activities for counselors: Harnessing solutions to common problems* (pp. 251–256). New York: Taylor & Francis.

Green, S., & Bobele, M. (1988). An interactional approach to marital infidelity: Including the other woman in therapy. *Journal of Strategic and Systemic Therapies*, *7*(4), 35–47.

Green, S., & Flemons, D. (Eds.). (2007). *Quickies: The handbook of brief sex therapy* (1st ed.). New York: Norton.

Green, S., & Flemons, D. (Eds.). (2018). *Quickies: The handbook of brief sex therapy* (3rd ed.). New York: Norton.

Green, S., Rolleston, M., & Schroeder, M. (2018). Equine assisted therapy with couples and families in crisis. In K. S. Trotter & J. Baggerly (Eds.). *Equine assisted therapy activities for counselors: Harnessing solutions to common problems* (pp. 238–248). New York: Taylor & Francis.

Green, S., Schroeder, M., Rolleston, M., Penalva, C., & Judd, V. (2018). Triggering transformations: An equine assisted approach to the treatment of substance abuse. In K. S. Trotter & J. Baggerly (Eds.). *Equine assisted therapy activities for counselors: Harnessing solutions to common problems* (pp. 161–168). New York: Taylor & Francis.

Selvini Palazzoli, M., Cecchin, G., Prata, G., & Boscolo, L. (1978). *Paradox and counterparadox: A new model in the therapy of the family in schizophrenic transaction.* New York: Jason Aronson.

Watzalwick, P., Weakland, P., & Fisch, R. (1974). *Change: Principles of problem formation and problem resolution.* New York: Norton.

CHAPTER 10

Going "One-Down"[1]

Michael F. Hoyt

The strategic therapy tactic of taking a "one-down position" was described by Richard Fisch, John Weakland, and Lynn Segal (1982) in their classic book *The Tactics of Change: Doing Therapy Briefly*. The key idea, which they discussed under the rubric of "therapist maneuverability," involves minimizing resistance and exerting influence by appearing modest or humble. As Gilbert Greene (1996, p. 133) explained: "In the treatment situation the clinician is inherently in a one-up, authority position and the client feels in a one-down position by the very nature of having a problem necessitating professional help. Such an arrangement may increase client resistance and decrease cooperation since people often resent experts and authorities (Fisch et al., 1982), especially when feeling one-down. In order to counter this barrier, it is helpful for the clinician to take a *one-down position*. The one-down position is often subtly conveyed and can be expressed in a variety of ways." As I'll discuss in what follows, some of these ways can produce a surprised, *You Said What?* response.

The ideas of "playing dumb" and "leading from behind" are not new or limited to psychotherapy, of course. "Make your victims feel smart – seem dumber than your mark" is the way Robert Greene (1998, p. 145–155) put it in *The 48 Laws of Power*. Examples might include TV's Lieutenant Columbo (played by Peter Falk), who would ask seemingly bumbling questions until the suspects' answers revealed their crimes; Langston Hughes' (1965) *Simple's Uncle Sam* and various "wise fool" spiritual traditions (see Buber, 1947; Reps, 1957; Shah, 1969); as well as Muhammed Ali's "rope-a-dope" strategy, in which he let a boxing opponent flail away at him harmlessly until the opponent was tired and ready to be K.O.'d.

My purpose here is to illustrate and stimulate some ideas about how and when to use a "one-down" position. Before recounting some clinical episodes, however, I would like to describe three situations from my professional developmental path, two from long ago and one more mid-career, in which taking "one-down" positions proved advantageous in helping me – not a client – to achieve a goal. In these episodes, "one-downsmanship" was a maneuver used in the face of strong countervailing forces. I offer them in the hope that readers will find various implications for their own situations. It's not always easier or wise to ride a horse in the direction it's going (e.g., when it's running toward a low branch or a cliff), and you don't want to get tossed or run over, either!

Three Non-Clinical Instances of Going "One-Down"

Instance #1. Before starting graduate school, in 1970–71 I took a year off as I waited for my girlfriend to finish college. Among my part-time jobs, I was working at the UCLA Psychology Department as a proofreader for the *Journal of Social Issues (JSI)*. Arthur R. Jensen (1969) had recently published his very controversial paper, "How Much Can We Boost IQ and Scholastic Achievement?" in the *Harvard Educational Review*. Jensen, a professor at the University of California-Berkeley, was a major proponent of the hereditarian position in the nature and nurture debate, the position that genetics play a significant role in behavioral traits, such as intelligence and personality. His paper concluded, among other things, that Head Start programs designed to boost African-Americans' IQ scores had failed, and that this was likely never to be remedied, largely because, in Jensen's estimation, 80% of the variance in IQ in the population studied was the result of genetic factors and the remainder was due to environmental influences.

The paper initiated a firestorm, and the *JSI* was planning a special issue on the topic. Dr. Raven, the journal editor, wasn't there when Professor Jensen called to speak to him. I answered the phone and took a message to have the editor call Professor Jensen. Before hanging up, I asked:

> "Dr. Jensen, I'm just the journal proofreader here now, but I'm studying to be a psychologist and I read your very interesting paper. I have an analysis that I think is correct. Would you like to hear it?"
> "Well, OK ... sure."
> "It goes like this, sir. We captured these people and shackled them on ships, then tortured them in slavery for 300 years, then supposedly freed them, but many or most were kept in poverty. Their families were wrecked. Many still have poor nutrition and don't get prenatal care. They get the worst schools and teachers and lousy old books. Then we write the tests, based on our experience – and we still can only beat them on average by 3 or 4 or 5 points. Doesn't that suggest that they're really smarter than we are?"
> It was quiet on the other end.
> "Well, Dr. Jensen, what do you think? Is there anything I'm missing?"
> "Please have Professor Raven call me when he comes in."

When Dr. Raven came back from lunch, I told him that Professor Jensen had called. After he spoke with Jensen, he asked me what exactly I had said. I told him.

"You really said that to him?"

"Yeah."

He laughed, then said, "I don't think it was your place to challenge him."

I apologized for any trouble I might have caused, but added, "I'm right though, aren't I?"

He chuckled again. "Maybe – it's certainly a different interpretation. I wish I'd seen the look on his face."

Comment. In fairness to Dr. Jensen, he was an earnest scientist and later claimed that "the cause of the difference remains an open question." His work was cited more than 20 times in *The Bell Curve* (Herrnstein & Murray, 1994), however, a book that promulgated the view that IQ test differences were essentially indicative of white superiority; and he accepted more than $1 million in research funding from an organization known for its racist viewpoint.

Instance #2. In 1985 I got a call from Dr. Lewis ("Larry") Wolberg, who was then the Director of the Postgraduate Center for Mental Health, in New York; and the editor (1965) of *Short-Term Psychotherapy*, the first major book on the topic published in the U.S. He had just read my recently published paper, "Therapist Resistances to Short-Term Dynamic Psychotherapy" (1985) and invited me to participate in the 1986 conference they were going to hold in Puerto Vallarta, Mexico (near where he had his winter home).

I was the most junior and least experienced faculty member at the conference. The other faculty members included several persons who have gone on to become major leaders in psychology and psychiatry. They were all nice fellows, but when it came time for some clinical role-playing demonstrations they were all jostling for position, and I got pushed aside. "Sorry, Michael, but it looks like all the therapist roles are taken." I was feeling forlorn, then had an idea: "That's OK – I'll play the patient." And I did, with each rising star. Knowing a bit about their respective approaches and different theories of psychotherapy, I was a most difficult patient: The guy who wanted to write medication prescriptions had to deal with me wanting to talk about my mother and the meaning of life, the CBT specialist had to deal with me crying and declaring that I needed to talk to someone about having been abused and molested, and the psychodynamic and personality disorder specialist had someone on his hands complaining of dry mouth, tiredness, and decreased appetite and sleep! One down, but far from out! (Dr. Wolberg also invited me back to be a discussant at the next year's conference.)

Instance #3. In 2000, I was honored to be invited to be a keynote speaker at the First Pan-Pacific Brief Therapy Conference, held in Fukuoka, Japan. I presented my recently published paper, "A Golfer's Guide to Brief Therapy (with Footnotes for Baseball Fans)" (Hoyt, 2000/2017). Following the format of a golf course, the paper lays out 18 principles of brief therapy with supporting anecdotes from the sports worlds of golf and baseball. When my Japanese discussant offered his comments, he scolded me: "You are in Japan and should use Japanese examples, not ones from golf and baseball." He was perhaps right, although his tone was harsh – and some Japanese do play golf and they have a long tradition of baseball, including Babe Ruth playing there in 1934. He upbraided me, left and right. Finally, when it was my time to reply, I bowed deeply. "You are right, of course," I said, "and I would have known more if I had only listened better to my paper. Now I see." I then proceeded to carefully recite and review many of my points (e.g., Know where the hole is, Avoid resistance, Be efficient, Have a here-and-now orientation, Use local knowledge, Speak the client's language). When I finished, I bowed again.

Afterward, a colleague from Hong Kong introduced himself. "Michael," he said, "I knew you were smart. Now I think you are also wise!" Made my day.

Comment. My discussant's instruction also stayed with me. When I spoke the next time at a conference in Osaka, Japan, I started with a bow and modest apology for possibly boring the audience, recited haiku, called other presenters *sensei*, told the story of the three lords at the local castle, and quoted Ichiro Suzuki, the great Japanese baseball player – see Hoyt, 2001/2017. Later during the conference, I also saw another one-down maneuver. After another presenter gave a paper, an audience member asked a very, very long and involved interminable question, one that went on and on and mostly seemed to be a way of the questioner showing off. When he finally finished, the presenter simply asked, "I'm sorry – could you repeat the question?" Like in marital arts, thrown by his own weight![2]

And Now … On to Therapy

All communications are either symmetrical or complementary (Watzlawick et al., 1967, p. 70). In therapy it is usually the situation that the therapist is "up" and the client is "down," that is, the therapist is the expert and the client is the petitioner of the therapist's services. This is an example of a complementary relationship. It sometimes can be useful for the therapist to take a one-down position, however, to help elevate the client's sense of value and empowerment and to avoid the therapist being perceived as a threat if the client is feeling especially vulnerable and it appears that taking a one-up position will only escalate resistance and conflict. (Still a complementary relationship, but with the positions reversed.) To diminish the implied hierarchical distance between the therapist and the patient, Segal (2001, p. 90) recommended everyone using first names, the therapist portraying him or herself as another human being with frailties and limitations, the therapist saying "I'm one of those people who have to hear things about five times before I get it," advising the patient[3] to "go slow," and offering new ideas or directives as "not very important, just one small thing that might be of some help."

A lot can get done just by being respectful, curious, and non-arrogant. Consulting in the hospital with a medical-surgical patient who had undergone a total hip replacement, for example, I asked if I could get some advice: "I've never had this kind of surgery – I know each person is an individual, but is there any information or helpful hints you can give me that I can pass on to other people who have the same kind of operation? What would be good for them to know?" As the patient described various practical ways to manage pain, cope with boredom, and how to get up and around to use the toilet, the patient became The Expert, his knowledge transcending his individual experience and now benefiting others.

In what follows, I offer two other "going one-down" clinical examples (from Hoyt, 2017) because they involved somewhat more unusual behaviors.

Case Example #1. I was called to the Emergency Room to see a crisis patient who had been brought in by his family because of his anger, agitation, and potential violence. When I looked in I saw a large, upset, pacing, wide-eyed and somewhat frightening man. (I'm also tall and although I now look like a grandfather with a balky back, bald pate and a fringe of shaggy white hair and a goatee, in those days I was a lean competitive athlete and looked strong and alpha-male.) I didn't want to provoke a macho confrontation, so I sat in a wheelchair, leaned to one side, and had a nurse push me into the room and stay (silently) while I talked with the patient. Once he saw my situation, he calmed down – I think he may have even felt a bit sorry for me. He sat down, lowered his voice and asked me if I was OK, and we spoke without incident.

Comment: It is good to know your stimulus value, how you look and come across – and to make necessary adjustments for different situations in order for the relationship to work.

Case Example #2. In another situation (which also involved a wheelchair), I literally went one-down. Sam was an elderly man when I first met him sitting next to his wife in the waiting room of the HMO Psychiatry clinic. He had been referred by his internist: "Post-stroke. Fear of falling." When I introduced myself and we shook hands, I could see that he was a pleasant and engaging man. He had not shaved in a few days, was casually dressed, and was wearing an Oakland A's baseball cap. His wife immediately began to talk (a lot) and quickly told me that Sam could walk but was afraid to. He had come into the building on his own, and then gotten into the wheelchair. She was nice and trying to be helpful, but I sensed that it would be useful to have some time with the patient alone, so I asked: "Do you want to walk or ride to my office?" He replied: "I'll take a ride, at least this time."

As I pushed him around the corner and down the corridor, we talked baseball – about a recent trade and how the game had gone that day. His remarks showed a good knowledge of the game and an alert, up-to-date interest. I asked questions, and we connected as we talked.

At my office door I stopped and asked him to take a few steps into my office and use a regular chair, so that I would not have to move the furniture around – an indirect approach that used his natural courtesy to bypass discussion of his need for the wheelchair. He obliged. When we sat down, I learned that he was a retired mechanic and printing pressman. He had suffered a stroke three years earlier, with a residual partial paralysis of one arm and leg. He had grown "too damn dependent" on his wife, he said, but could no longer drive and had considerable difficulty walking. "I sure miss Dr. Jarrett," he interjected, referring to his former internist who had himself retired a few years earlier. I asked what Dr. Jarrett would have said to get him moving. When he told me, I "borrowed" the good doctor's mantle of authority and replied: "Took the words right out of my mouth."

Sam went on to tell me that he wanted to go to an upcoming game his sons had invited him to, but he had to first overcome his great fear of falling because "I get so worried and down that I freeze up." He knew how to fall safely (protecting his head and softening the fall) but was fearful because "I'm not sure what would happen to me if I fell and no one was around. I might not be able to get back up."

(By coincidence, I had the night before read my then young son a story [Peet, 1972] about a series of animals that each gets stranded, culminating with an elephant stuck on his back until an ant he had befriended rescues him with the help of an ant hoard.)

Sam was a practical man with a predicament. After ascertaining that he was not worried about safety or embarrassment, I suggested: "I'll tell you what. Let's do a little experiment. I'll be you, you be the coach, and teach me how to get up." I then proceeded to sort of throw myself on the floor in front of him. He got right into it, advising me, "No, turn the other way, get up first on three points," etc. I said, "Let's try it with my arm not working," and held it limply against my side. For the next several minutes I repeatedly got down on the floor and Sam instructed me on how to get myself up again.

Back in my chair, I asked him if he wanted to "try it" there in my office or wait until he got home – an "illusion of alternatives" (Watzlawick, 1978) with the underlying implication that he would perform the action. He chose to wait until he was home but offered to show me "some exercises I can still do." I watched and then asked him to "stand and do a little walking just so I can see how you do." I opened the office door and we proceeded into the corridor. We slowly made our way up and down the hallway, with my remarking a couple of times "Good" and "Nice, better than I expected." As we went up and down the hallway I switched back to baseball, asking him about the game he was planning to attend with his sons. "Where are you going to park? Which ramp will you take?" I painted aloud a vivid picture of father and sons entering the baseball stadium as we made our way up and down the hallway a couple of times.

Back in my office he expressed concern about his wife. She was trying to be helpful but was wearing out both herself and Sam with her watchfulness. "Maybe you could talk to her, too?" he asked. I said I would be glad to "when you begin to do more walking on your own so that I'll really be able to convince her to back off." He understood and agreed to practice his falling and getting up, and we playfully bargained about how many times he would do it a day, letting him "win" the negotiation and settling on twice a day to start and then three times a day until I saw him in two weeks.

Before leaving my office, I added, "You know, I think it's really important that you go to that game with your sons if you can. I know you want to, but I think it will be even more important for them. Someday they will look back and remember going to the game with you, you know what I mean?" Sam did not know exactly how baseball was in my blood, my history of going to games with my father, but he knew I was saying something heartfelt and important. It spoke to him. "I'm sure going to give it my best," he said. "Dr. Jarrett would like that," I replied.

Comment. There is more to this story, of course – see Hoyt, 2017, pp. 62–65. Suffice it to say, Sam achieved his goals. The point here is that it was helpful and felt natural to temporarily reverse roles, Sam becoming the teacher/coach rather than the humbled stroke patient. This was morale-restoring and opened possibilities for change. Being alert to and structuring the therapeutic relationship as we did helped restore his confidence. My taking a one-down position and using whatever resources were available in the service of the patient's therapeutic needs – including my own personal experiences with baseball, inverted elephants, and father-son relations – is what I take Milton Erickson and Ernest Rossi (1979, p. 276) to have meant when they suggested: "To initiate this type of therapy you have to be yourself as a person. You cannot imitate somebody else, but you have to do it your own way."

When to Go One-Down – and What It Can Cost

A certain amount of humility is a form of courteous modesty ("Help me understand…"), an attitude and display of politeness and respect, and can also serve to lower unrealistic expectations. "One-downsmanship" becomes a therapeutic tactic when employed to encourage others, but can also be used disingenuously to actually be "one-up" as in the three non-clinical instances I described earlier in this chapter.

The idea of "therapist maneuverability" (Fisch et al., 1982) is not new or unique, of course. Franz Alexander and Thomas French (1946) suggested that therapists change their demeanor and stance (e.g., being indulgent versus strict) to help produce a "corrective emotional experience" with the particular patient. Arnold Lazarus (1993) counseled that the therapist should be an "authentic chameleon." In *Words Were Originally Magic*, Steve de Shazer (1994) described different ways of relating to clients. He contrasted Milton Erickson's "expert" stance with other, less hierarchical and more egalitarian positions, including what he called "de Shazer-the-stupid." He went on (p. 34) to add: "Actually, I should have seen all of this long ago, since the two major influences on my interviewing style have been John Weakland's persona 'Weakland-the-dense' and Insoo Kim Berg's persona 'Insoo-the-incredulous.'" (Insoo was Steve's wife, by the way.) Those of us who knew Steve and John and Insoo (see

Hoyt & Berg, 1998; Hoyt, 2012/2015), even as we recall Insoo often exclaiming "Wow! How did you do that?" with seeming amazement in her voice, appreciate how very "non-dense" and brilliant they were.

Operating from the assumption that "the client is the expert" (Anderson & Goolishian, 1992) can facilitate client empowerment, but can also reduce what social psychologists call "communicator credibility" (Hovland, Janis, & Kelley, 1953) – the "common factors" (Duncan et al., 2010) belief in the therapist which may foster confidence and contribute to a positive therapeutic alliance and favorable outcomes. Clients who are used to being "boss" (by dint of hard work, age, occupational position, or other factors) may find it more congenial to be "one-up." There are also clients (perhaps especially from some cultural groups) who may want and expect the therapist to be an expert and will not be pleased or respect a clinician who avoids being one-up. They are seeking help from a professional, and don't want a klutz and don't want to feel patronized. Thus, Don Meichenbaum (2013, p. 202), in discussing the "Art of Questioning," endorses emulating Lt. Columbo, but also goes on to caution that too much of a one-down position can undermine the therapist's credibility and useful authority: "I encourage clinicians to 'play dumb,' using their befuddlement, confusion, and Socratic questioning style. For some clinicians, of course, 'playing dumb' comes naturally. The trick is how to be inquisitive, without giving up your 'placebo value.'"

Indeed: that is part of the art and craft of communication. Done right, taking a "one-down" position can evoke resources, surprise, and appreciation.

Notes

1 Case Example #2 ("Sam") originally appeared in M.F. Hoyt (2009), *Brief Psychotherapies: Principles and Practices*. Phoenix, AZ: Zeig, Tucker & Theisen. ©M.F. Hoyt 2009. Used with permission.

2 Or, as Shakespeare said (*Hamlet*, Act III, Scene iv, line 207), "Hoist with his own petard." (A *petard* was a bomb, so meaning "blown up with his own device.") In these examples (especially with the windbag questioner and the sharp-elbowed colleagues), going "one-down" was not used therapeutically to elevate the other, but rather, with some passive-aggression, to advance one's own position. *Touché!*

3 The term *client* was popularized by Carl Rogers (1951) as an alternative to *patient* partially as a way of reducing hierarchy – *patient* evokes a medical model with images of a sick person seeking help from a wise doctor; whereas *client* may seem more humanistic and egalitarian (Hoyt, 1979/2017).

References

Alexander, F. & French, T.M. (1946). *Psychoanalytic therapy: Theory and applications.* New York: Ronald Press.

Anderson, H., & Goolishian, H.A. (1992). The client is the expert: A not-knowing approach to therapy. In S. McNamee & K.J. Gergen (Eds.). *Therapy as social construction* (pp. 25–39). Newbury Park, CA: Sage.

Buber, M. (1947). *Tales of the Hasidim (Vol. 1, The early masters; Vol. 2, The late masters).* New York: Schocken Books.

de Shazer, S. (1994). *Words were originally magic.* New York: Norton.

Duncan, B.L., Miller, S.D., Wampold, B.E., & Hubble, M.A. (Eds.). (2010). *The heart and soul of change: Delivering what works in therapy* (2nd ed.). Washington, DC: APA Books.

Erickson, M.H., & Rossi, E.L. (1979). *Hypnotherapy: An exploratory casebook.* New York: Irvington.

Fisch, R., Weakland, J.H., & Segal, L. (1982). *The tactics of change: Doing therapy briefly.* San Francisco: Jossey-Bass.

Greene, G.J. (1996). Communication theory and social work treatment. In F.J. Turner (Ed.). *Social work treatment: Interlocking theoretical approaches* (4th ed., pp. 116–145). New York: Free Press/Simon & Schuster.

Greene, R. (1998). *The 48 laws of power.* New York: Penguin.

Herrnstein, R.J., & Murray, C. (1994). *The Bell curve: Intelligence and class structure in American life.* New York: Free Press/Simon & Schuster.

Hovland, C.I., Janis, I.L., & Kelley, H.H. (1953). *Communication and persuasion.* New Haven, CT: Yale University Press.

Hoyt, M.F. (1979). "Patient" or "client": What's in a name? *Psychotherapy: Theory, Research, and Practice, 16,* 46–47. Reprinted in M.F. Hoyt, *Brief therapy and beyond* (pp. 1–2). New York: Routledge, 2017.

Hoyt, M.F. (1985). Therapist resistances to short-term dynamic psychotherapy. *Journal of the American Academy of Psychoanalysis, 13,* 93–112. Reprinted in M.F. Hoyt, *Brief therapy and managed care: Readings for contemporary practice* (pp. 219-235). San Francisco: Jossey-Bass, 1995.

Hoyt, M.F. (2000). A golfer's guide to brief therapy (with footnotes for baseball fans). In *Some stories are better than others: Doing what works in brief therapy and managed care* (pp. 5–15). New York: Brunner/Mazel. Reprinted in M.F. Hoyt, *Brief therapy and beyond: Stories, language, love, hope, and time* (pp. 33–43). New York: Routledge, 2017.

Hoyt, M.F. (2001). *Toward a more effective brief therapy.* Keynote speech, Second Pan-Pacific Brief Therapy Conference, Osaka, Japan. Reprinted in M.F. Hoyt, *Brief therapy and beyond: Stories, language, love, hope, and time* (pp. 204–210). New York: Routledge, 2017.

Hoyt, M.F. (2012). Remembering Steve de Shazer and Insoo Kim Berg. In M. Vogt, F. Wolf, P. Sundman, & H.N. Dreesen (Eds.). *Meeting Steve de Shazer and Insoo Kim Berg* [in German; pp. 73–77]. Dortmund, Germany: Verlag ModerneLernen/Borgmann Publishers. Reprinted in English as *Encounters with Steve de Shazer and Insoo Kim Berg* (pp. 76–80). London: Solutions Books, 2015.

Hoyt, M.F., & Berg, I.K. (1998). Solution-focused couple therapy: Helping clients construct self-fulfilling prophecies. In M.F. Hoyt (Ed.). *The handbook of constructive therapies* (pp. 314–340). San Francisco: Jossey-Bass.

Hughes, L. (1965). *Simple's Uncle Sam.* New York: Hill and Wang.

Jensen, A.C. (1969). How much can we boost IQ and scholastic achievement? *Harvard Educational Review, 39,* 1–123.

Lazarus, A.A. (1993). Tailoring the therapeutic relationship, or being an authentic chameleon. *Psychotherapy: Theory, Research, & Practice, 30*(3), 404–407.

Meichenbaum, D. (2013). At my mother's kitchen table: Who are we, but the stories we tell? In M.F. Hoyt (Ed.), *Therapist stories of inspiration, passion, and renewal: What's love got to do with it?* (pp. 195–205). New York: Routledge.

Peet, B. (1972). *The ant and the elephant.* Boston: Houghton Mifflin.

Reps, P. (1957). *Zen flesh, Zen bones: A collection of Zen and pre-Zen writings.* North Clarendon, VT: Tuttle Publishing.

Rogers, C. (1951). *Client-centered therapy.* Boston: Houghton Mifflin.

Segal, L. (2001). Brief therapy. In R.J. Corsini (Ed.). *Handbook of innovative therapy* (2nd ed., pp. 86–94). New York: Wiley.

Shah, I. (1969). *Wisdom of the idiots.* London: Octagon Press.

Watzlawick, P. (1978). *The language of change: Elements of therapeutic communication.* New York: Norton.

Watzlawick, P., Beavin, J. H., & Jackson, D.D. (1967). *Pragmatics of human communication: A study of interactional patterns, pathologies, and paradoxes.* New York: Norton.

Wolberg, L.R. (Ed.) (1965). *Short-term psychotherapy.* Philadelphia: Grune & Stratton.

CHAPTER 11

"No Way – You Gotta Be Kidding!"
Using Ordeals to Promote Problem-Stopping[1]

Michael F. Hoyt

My usual therapy approach, rooted in narrative constructivism, is to assist people in making desired changes by helping them alter what they are telling themselves about themselves, other people, and their situations (Hoyt, 2017). Sometimes, however, there is a particular behavior that needs to be stopped, and "re-storying" is just too slow or not effective. At such times, a useful strategic intervention[2] can be enlisting the client's full cooperation and then prescribing an ordeal. As Jay Haley (1984, p. 5) wrote in *Ordeal Therapy: Unusual Ways to Change Behavior*: "If one makes it more difficult for a person to have a symptom than give it up, the person will give up the symptom."

Ordeal Therapy was one of Haley's finest books. Written with his typical clarity, full of humor and shorn of obfuscating jargon, Haley (1984, p. xi) explained: "This is a book about the absurd dilemmas people find themselves in and the absurd solutions offered them in therapy." In the book's Introduction, Haley quoted Erickson's description of his famous case of a man with insomnia who was given the task of polishing the floor all night if he wasn't asleep within 15 minutes – the man soon chose the "lesser of two evils" and was sleeping soundly throughout the night! (Viewers of the 1993 Haley and Richeport videotape can watch Erickson tell the story himself.)

Haley (1984, pp. 6–7) outlined the ordeal technique:

> With the ordeal technique, the therapist's task is easily defined: It is to impose an ordeal appropriate to the problem of the person who wants to change, an ordeal more severe than the problem. The main requirement of an ordeal is that it cause distress equal to, or greater than, that caused by the symptom, just as a punishment should fit the crime. Usually, if an ordeal isn't severe enough to extinguish the symptom, it can be increased in magnitude until it is. It is also best if the ordeal is good for the person. Doing what's good for you is hard for anyone and seems particularly difficult for people who seek therapy... One final aspect of the ordeal:

Sometimes the person must go through it repeatedly to recover from the symptom. At other times the mere threat of an ordeal brings recovery. That is, when the therapist lays out the ordeal as a procedure and the person agrees to experience it, he or she often abandons the symptom before the ordeal even goes into effect.

Haley then described different types of ordeals:

1. *Straightforward Tasks*, such as having a person exercise, preferably in the middle of the night, each time the problem occurs. He emphasized the importance of securing the patient's ironclad agreement to do the task, and commented that "the exercise should be sufficient so that it can be felt in the muscles the next day" (p. 10).
2. *Paradoxical Ordeals*, for example, having a depressed patient schedule specific times to be depressed, directing a phobic patient to imagine repeatedly that which he or she fears, or requiring a quarreling couple to quarrel. "It is a question whether a paradoxical intervention can be anything but an ordeal insofar as individuals are asked to go through what they'd rather recover from" (p. 10).
3. *The Therapist as an Ordeal*, including interventions in which the therapist reframes, confronts, or interprets the patient's behavior such that the patient is forced to face or think about the problem in ways they would rather avoid.[3]
4. *Ordeals Involving Two or More Persons*, for instance, having a mother check a child's bed at dawn and, if the bed is wet, having her help him practice handwriting (or, I might add, having the father wash the sheets, which would involve him in the triangle and probably create an ordeal they would rather avoid).[4]

Haley (1984, pp. 12–13) also cautioned that while the therapist should provide an ordeal that the person would choose to avoid by giving up the symptomatic behavior, ordeals should be benevolent and not be used as a method of social control or for persecution of the public under the guise of therapy. Burns (2001) reminds us that Haley also wrote in *Uncommon Therapy* (1973, p. 25) about "providing a worse alternative." O'Hanlon (1987, pp. 43–48) referred to ordeals as "symptom-contingent tasks." Short et al. (2005, p. 203) considered ordeals as a class of double-binds, citing another Erickson case of a man with insomnia wherein "Erickson established a contingency [standing and reading all night if not sleeping] that enabled the man to punish himself constructively any time he wanted." In my words, we erect an impediment that makes the problematic behavior not worth continuing. We don't quite "make them an offer they can't refuse," *à la The Godfather*, but we help patients to give up a symptom by offering them a chance to take an easier way out, "a path of less resistance."

Haley (1984) also outlined the stages of ordeal therapy:

1. The problem must be defined clearly.
2. The person must be committed to getting over the problem.
3. An ordeal must be selected.
4. The directive must be given with a rationale. "[The therapist] must make clear that the task is to occur only with symptomatic behavior and that there is a set time for it. Exactly what is to be done must be described. If appropriate, the task must be given with a rationale that makes it seem reasonable ... For some people, it is best to not explain but simply to tell them to do it. This more magical approach is best for the intellectuals among the clientele who can undo or explain away any rationale and find the whole thing not necessary" (pp. 15–16).
5. The ordeal continues until the problem is resolved.
6. The ordeal is in a social context. The therapist helps the client through the reorganization of the client's life.

In *Ordeal Therapy*, Haley (1984) presented a series of interesting, well-observed case reports. An ordeal was designed in each situation that served as an onerous burden that had to be performed by the patient if/when the problem behavior beckoned or occurred. Haley (and Erickson) would first get patients to give their word to do the task even before they knew what it actually entailed. He would tell them that it was not illegal or immoral, but that they must promise to do whatever it was. He said that under those conditions – which Watzlawick, Weakland, and Fisch (1974, p. 154–157) called a "Devil's Pact" – he could help the person. He would get them to make a promise that locked them in. For example, in one instance a priest bothered by pleasant sexual sensations while showering agreed, in desperation, to do whatever the therapist recommended – and was then instructed to take repeated showers, sometimes for many hours a day. In another case, a competent man who said that he wanted to do more but was just spending all his days sitting passively was led to agree to shave off his luxuriant moustache, his one source of pride, if he didn't begin to work – and so he began active employment. In another case, in which Milton Erickson was the therapist, a woman enmeshed with an adult schizophrenic son was induced to drop him off for long walks in the Arizona desert. In yet another instance, an artist prone to becoming a derelict bum needed the ordeal of "hitting bottom" to trigger his taking a healthier path. A 17-year-old bed-wetter, if he awoke in a wet bed, would have to go for a long night walk, then return and climb back into the wet bed. A man not asleep by a certain time would have to stand and read all night. Other ordeals were created to deal with a disputatious couple with screaming toddlers, a teenage set of identical twins having difficulty differentiating, a 10-year-old boy with compulsive public masturbation, parents with a pants-pooping 5-year-old boy, a woman with compulsive hand-washing, another woman with binge-purge vomiting, another set of parents with an 8-year-old having major temper tan-trums, a woman who wanted a partner but avoided dating, and other challeng-ing situations.

Haley's full descriptions merit careful study to enjoy the subtleties of the strategies and artful clinical interaction, including various nuances and adjustments. The therapies were successful. Problems were defined, the clients' cooperation secured, an ordeal selected and presented in a way that gained the clients' compliance, the ordeal was continued until the problem was resolved, and the ordeal and desired solution were integrated into the social context of the clients' life.

Ordeal Therapy Today

The theory and techniques of ordeal therapy – making it too hard (or at least, not worth it) to continue a problematic behavior – are still relevant, of course, although in today's therapy climate (doctors seen less as Ultimate Authority figures, elaborate informed-consent procedures,[5] an overemphasis on medica-tions and cognitive-behavioral interventions rather than systemic and inter-actional approaches, etc.) therapists might have more difficulty getting clients to comply with some of the ordeals that Erickson and Haley constructed. Still, the very hassle of dealing with insurance companies and HMO limits can be an ordeal in itself that may encourage some people not to dawdle but to resolve their problems as soon as possible (John Frykman, 2009, personal communication).

Sometimes just quoting to people the old saying "If you don't change direc-tions, you're going to wind up where you're heading!" is enough to make them expect an unending ordeal if they don't do something different. Other times, they may need a taste. A man consulted me for help because of dif-ficulty breaking off an affair. He had stopped seeing the paramour but was tempted to recontact her. We talked about the high probability of getting caught, his wife's inevitable angry recriminations, paying for unsuccessful marriage counseling, divorce, endless alimony and child support, and hav-ing to move from his house to a small condo somewhere. The specter of these consequences raised his anxiety, but he was still sorely tempted. What really made the difference, I think, was when I persuaded him that each time he felt the urge to call his old girlfriend, he should go, *"since that may be where you're heading anyway,"* on Sunday morning to the local pancake house to observe all the divorced fathers and less-than-happy kids having breakfast before end-ing their weekend visitations and returning to mom. He did go, that Sunday, and reported to me what he had noticed: "A lot of the dads and kids looked miserable. It was terrible. I'll do anything not to have to do that again." He ended the affair.

Another time (reported in Hoyt, 1995/2017) a woman with bridge phobia (no small problem for someone living in the San Francisco Bay area, where

I practice) came to see me. Since she wanted the best treatment, I persuaded her that more data would be necessary about her reactions at different times and locations, and so under my direction she began driving – sometimes quite anxiously – across several bridges at varying times of day and night. This experiment promoted both her desensitizing exposure and convinced her that she could drive with reasonable comfort as long as she could avoid the ordeal of rush-hour traffic.

In another instance, my wife and I were once sitting in a marriage counselor's office spending $100 an hour arguing about whether to spend $50 a week on a housecleaner – I did the math, *cha-ching!* and realized how to end the ordeal.

Here's another example: A man and woman who had heard about my interest in couple therapy (see Hoyt, 2015) sought me out. They said that they wanted to spend more enjoyable time together, but they repeatedly were "too busy" to keep the dates they planned. We discussed communication and commitment. There were promises but nothing changed. After a few rounds of "Yes, buts" and "No, buts," I said, "I'm not helping. I don't think we should keep meeting." They protested they were desperate and would do anything.

"*Anything?*" I asked (my mind rising Haleyesque).

"Yes. We really love one another and don't want to ruin our relationship."

"I'm sorry. I'd like to help – but I don't think you're really ready to change."

"We are!" (They had pledged their compliance quickly – perhaps too quickly – so I pressed them a bit to really set the hook.)

"I hear what you're saying, but I'm not sure. You know, actions speak louder than words."

"Please help us. We'll do anything."

I knew they were both politically active. They were wearing campaign buttons and had made references to attending meetings and rallies. Indeed, they were spending a great deal of time working for a certain candidate – so much time that they didn't have much left to be a couple.

"Well, other than breaking up, what would be something really bad that you really don't want to see happen?"

They looked at one another, then both quickly said they would hate to see their candidate's opponent win.

"Well then, if you'll do exactly what I say, I think I can help you." I paused for effect, then continued: "Before I'll tell you, though, you have to swear on your honor, on the Bible, on your love, and on any future unborn child's head that you'll do it, whatever I say. I promise it won't be illegal." (The hyperbole was to make what followed humorous and palatable – see Hoyt & Andreas, 2015; the reference to a future child was intended to appeal to what might be at stake.)

They looked at one another, then assented: "OK. We'll do it. What?"

"Are you sure?"

"Yeah."

"First, let's shake hands on your word."

We shook.

"OK. What is it?"

"You have to agree to make a financial contribution to _____ (the hated candidate) if you don't go out together and spend the money on something enjoyable."

The man looked at me. "No way – you gotta be kidding!"

"No, I'm serious. I don't like _____ either, but this is therapy. It's time to fish or cut bait. You have to let me hold two $20 bills with the understanding that I will mail it to _____ if you don't go out on a date and have a good time. No ifs, ands, or buts." I took an envelope out of my desk, wrote the hated candidate's name on it, and held out my hand: "Your money or your lives."

They laughed. "It's a deal. No way is _____ ever gonna get our money!"

I don't know if they lived happily ever after, but I do know they went on a date, and then another and another. When I saw them last, they said that they were still working for their candidate and were continuing to make time for each other and were happy. I took the envelope out of my desk and gave them back their money.

Cautions and Conclusion

Perhaps obvious to say, but worth remembering: do no harm – don't impose an ordeal that may hurt the person, don't encourage addiction or violence. To have success, the clinician needs to assure, as much as possible, compliance that the patient will do the ordeal – several of Erickson's rare unsuccessful cases (see Hoyt, 2000) seem to be attributable to patients not following through on directives Erickson had given. Battino and South (2005) cautioned that the main problem in ordeal therapy is how to "hook" the client. They've got to feel obligated to undergo the ordeal if they do the problem – they've got to really feel that stopping the problem is the only way to avoid the ordeal. If trying to disrupt a problem pattern by adding an ordeal element, make sure the client is desperate enough that they'll agree to do the ordeal. For some people, of course, what Einstein called a *Gedankenexperiment* ("thought experiment") may be adequate – someone may just need the idea and not have to do the actual ordeal.

It is also important to be culturally sensitive. One wants an ordeal that clients would change their behavior to avoid, but not something offensive or destructive – don't suggest sending clients' money to the Nazis or the Ku Klux Klan. It is almost always better, as with the successful couple described above, to have them specify their own ordeal.

Good judgment and clinical skill are important. Haley and Erickson both had a sharp sense of irony and a great twinkle in their eyes. As quoted in

Crenshaw (2004, p. 46), when asked how he knew to use a certain intervention at a certain time, Jay replied: "You wouldn't use it on someone it wouldn't work on!"

Notes

1 Portions of this chapter are from Hoyt (2010) and used by agreement with Routledge (Taylor & Francis).
2 "Therapy can be called strategic if the clinician initiates what happens during therapy and designs a particular approach for each problem."—Haley (1973, p. 1)
3 Haley (1984, pp. 19–23) made clear that *ordeal* could be thought of as a theory of change, not just a technique limited to one approach. He noted that psychodynamic therapies involve the bringing forth of repressed, unpleasant material; that approaches derived from learning theory require giving up and changing reinforcements; and that systemic theories based on notions of homeostasis require new, often less-preferred behaviors. In his wry manner he also opined (p. 20): "Another characteristic of theories of change is that they must be conceptualized in such a way that they cannot be disproved. It is the theory no one can disprove, like the theory of the existence of God, that has a fair chance of living forever, if there is money in it."
4 Madanes (2006, p. 66) notes: "Interactional ordeals are particularly interesting. An ordeal could be for a husband to give his wife, or better yet his mother-in-law, a present every time the undesirable behavior occurs. The ordeal is something that the person dislikes but that would improve his relationship with significant others."
5 When I asked Paul Watzlawick (Hoyt, 1998/2001, p. 154), "From your frame, how do you think about *informed consent*?" he answered: "My 'informed consent' is the question: 'The next time you find yourself in the problem situation, would you be willing to carry out an experiment, namely to …?'"

References

Battino, R., & South, T.L. (2005). *Ericksonian approaches: A comprehensive manual* (2nd ed.). Bethel, CT: Crown House Publishing.

Burns, G. W. (2001). Jay Haley: The man who made therapy an ordeal. In J.K. Zeig (Ed.). *Changing directives: The strategic therapy of Jay Haley* (pp. 154–170). Phoenix, AZ: The Milton H. Erickson Foundation Press.

Crenshaw, W. (2004). *Treating families and children in the child protective system.* New York: Brunner-Routledge.

Haley, J. (1973). *Uncommon therapy: The psychiatric techniques of Milton H. Erickson, M.D.* New York: Norton.

Haley, J. (1984). *Ordeal therapy: Unusual ways to change behavior.* San Francisco: Jossey-Bass.

Haley, J., & Richeport, M. (1993). *Milton H. Erickson, M.D.: Explorer in hypnosis and therapy.* (videotape). New York: Brunner-Mazel.

Hoyt, M.F. (1995). Managed care, HMOs, and the Ericksonian perspective. *Ericksonian Monographs*, 1995, *10*, 25–36. Reprinted in M.F. Hoyt (2017), *Brief therapy and beyond: Stories, language, love, hope, and time* (pp. 44–69). New York: Routledge, 2017.

Hoyt, M.F. (1998). Constructing therapeutic realities: A conversation with Paul Watzlawick. In M.F. Hoyt (Ed.). *The handbook of constructive therapies* (pp. 183–197). San Francisco: Jossey-Bass. Reprinted in M.F. Hoyt, *Interviews with brief therapy experts* (pp. 144–157). New York: Brunner-Routledge, 2001.

Hoyt, M.F. (2000). What can we learn from Milton Erickson's therapeutic failures? In *Some stories are better than others: Doing what works in brief therapy and managed care* (pp. 189–194). New York: Brunner/Mazel.

Hoyt, M.F. (2010). Introduction—"An ordeal for pleasure: A story." In M. Richeport-Haley & J. Carlson (Eds.). *Jay Haley revisited* (pp. 49–74). New York: Routledge.

Hoyt, M.F. (2015). Solution-focused couple therapy. In A.S. Gurman, J.L. Lebow, & D. Snyder (Eds.), *Clinical handbook of couple therapy* (5th ed., pp. 300–332). New York: Guilford Press.

Hoyt, M.F. (2017). *Brief therapy and beyond: Stories, language, love, hope, and time.* New York: Routledge.

Hoyt, M.F., & Andreas, S. (2015). Humor in brief therapy: A dialogue. *Journal of Systemic Therapies, 34*(3), 13–24.

Madanes, C. (2006). Strategies and metaphors of brief therapy. In *The therapist as humanist, social activist, and systemic thinker ... and other selected papers* (pp. 62–78). Phoenix, AZ: Zeg, Tucker, & Theisen.

O'Hanlon, W.H. (1987). *Taproots: Underlying principles of Milton Erickson's therapy and hypnosis.* New York: Norton.

Short, D., Erickson, B.A., & Klein, R.E. (2005). *Hope and resiliency: Understanding the. psychotherapeutic strategies of Milton H. Erickson, M.D.* Norwalk, CT: Crown House Publishing.

Watzlawick, P., Weakland, J.H., & Fisch, R. (1974). *Change: Principles of problem formation and problem resolution.* New York: Norton.

CHAPTER 12

However Great the Question, It's the Answer That Makes a Difference

Chris Iveson

My professional world, the world of Solution-Focused Brief Therapy, is a topsy-turvy world where success still depends on trust – but on the therapist trusting the client rather than the other way around. Expertise is also crucial – however, it is the client's expertise, not the therapist's, that counts. Instead of the therapist understanding and solving problems, we have developed a conversational process which draws out and relies entirely on the clients' knowledge to create new possibilities for their lives. Taking the radical position that we cannot know (or prescribe) the "right" way forward for our clients, we have to trust their knowledge and treat them as the only experts in their own lives. We do this by establishing the client's desired outcome from our work together, not so much a goal, but a more encompassing "preferred future," or way of living where goals and other aspirations might be realized. We elicit a detailed description of how an outcome might manifest itself in the routine of the client's everyday life, and then trawl the past and present for the antecedents of this desired outcome. In other words, we invite clients to describe the future they are seeking and then look back from this point to discover the future's history. It is these detailed descriptions of possible futures and successful pasts that so often lead to the rapid and lasting changes associated with this model (Gingerich & Peterson, 2013; Ratner, George, & Iveson, 2012; Shennan & Iveson, 2011).

Case #1: The Empty Space: A "Fantastic" Couple

Joseph was described as a "revolving door schizophrenic," a characterization that carried little hope for his future well-being. He was referred by Donna, a community psychiatrist who had attended a short course at BRIEF, the center for Solution-Focused practice, founded by my two colleagues, Evan George and Harvey Ratner, and me. Though BRIEF is a private clinic we offer most of our therapy time free (our funding comes from training) so we are able to see those clients in extreme need for whom public-health services have proved inadequate. Donna had been very skeptical but was intrigued enough to bring a client to see us who so far had not responded to any treatment.

Joseph was a very jolly man and member of a "celebrity" family. From his late teens to his early 40s, he had been in and out of psychiatric hospitals and had made numerous suicide attempts, some very serious. Sitting at ease in our clinic, he was happy to tell me all his history. Listening to his sometimes harrowing tale I began to see a man of great personal strength and resourcefulness hidden behind the man most professionals had written off. Through Joseph's account of a seemingly failed life there began to appear a "shadow story" of survival, struggle, determination, perseverance, and hope. To hear this story, to read between the lines of what was being said, required of me a very intense form of listening verified by the occasional question, for example:

Chris: Could I just check, Joseph? On that last occasion when you so much wanted to die but then woke up back in hospital and not just any hospital but the one you most dread – how on earth did you begin to put the pieces of your life back together?

Questions like this clearly demonstrated attentive listening but were already beginning to invite Joseph to see another way of viewing his life story. When Joseph had finished his account, I was able to ask my usual opening question:

Chris: What are your best hopes from our talking together?

Joseph: I don't know, my social worker told me to come.

Chris: And if coming here proves to be a good idea, what difference do you hope it will make?

Joseph: To be honest, I don't really expect it to make a difference – nothing has.

Chris: If it did?

Joseph: If it did! Then I'd be able to get on and lead a normal life, get a job, get married.

At this point Joseph took a long look at the empty space to his right then turned back to me with a hopeless shrug saying,

Joseph: She's angry. She didn't want me to come here.

Not wanting to step into this strange territory without more familiarity with its contours, I sought to confirm with Joseph his desired outcome:

Chris: So, if our talking together led in some way to you leading a normal life, getting a job and possibly even getting married, would that mean it had been worthwhile?

Joseph: Yes. *(then turning again to the empty space on his right)* What do you think, Jenny?

Chris: If a miracle happened tonight while you were asleep, and it set your life on track towards a normal life with a job and a wife, what might be the first thing you'd notice?

Joseph: (turning to his right) She wouldn't tell me to kill myself.

Chris: What would she do instead?

Joseph: She'd agree to marry me! *(a laugh and, turning to his right, saying to the empty space)* You don't have to marry me if you don't want to.

This "three-way" conversation continued for a few minutes, with Joseph more often than not putting my questions to the silent and invisible "Jenny" whose answers, if she gave any, I was unable to hear. The "rule of thumb" in Solution-Focused practice is to ignore unusual or inexplicable behavior (provided no risk of harm is involved) and carry on asking the questions while listening for those answers (or fragments of answers) that can be built upon with further questions. This makes it perfectly possible to work successfully with clients under the influence of drugs or alcohol, or clients who are psychotic (but still prepared to answer questions) or suffering physical conditions such as Alzheimer's Disease. However, in this case Joseph's responses were problematic, as it is the client's answers that carry the possibility for change. Our job is to ask questions that the client hasn't been asked before, in order for them to say things they have never said before. These new ways of describing their world are what we believe leads to change. With Joseph not answering the questions, nothing useful was likely to come from our meeting.

Luckily, I was familiar with the work of Karl Tomm, one of the leading figures of family therapy (Tomm et al., 1998), especially his concept of "internalized others," a particularly creative take on the notion of multiple personalities. In a nutshell, Tomm puts forward a theory of personality based on our internalization of everyone we have met, and these people in some way reside within us and can be "retrieved." We can ask a person to *be* one of these others in order to elicit their perspectives on the person before us.

It was a "safe bet" that Jenny was one of Joseph's internalized others who had "escaped" or, to use the jargon, become "dissociated" from Joseph, her "host." But how to deal with this, here and now, in the session? My professional "upbringing" had been very clear on the notion of "collusion" with a client's view of the world – it was definitely not done. We were expected to challenge crazy ideas, not join in. Yet Solution-Focused practice requires us to work within the client's world because it is there that the necessary knowledge for a better life will be found. I had already been challenged many times in workshops for showing sessions with clients in which I had accepted (neither agreeing or disagreeing) their experiences as "real." Was what I was about to do next an "acceptance'" too far? I knew that the majority of mental-health professionals would, at that time, have been shocked by and even condemned what I was about to do, but in that moment I could see no other way forward so after a deep breath and with my heart in my mouth I asked:

Chris: Joseph, would you mind if I asked Jenny some questions?

Joseph: (looking to his right and then rather suspiciously at the therapist) Okay.

Chris: Obviously I can't see her, so will you be her for a few minutes?

Joseph: (looking a bit confused) Okay.

Chris: Jenny, what are your best hopes from this conversation?

Jenny (Joseph): I'd like Joseph to ignore me when I get angry and tell him to kill himself.

Chris: So, you don't really want him to kill himself?

Jenny (Joseph): Definitely not!

Chris: How come?

Jenny (Joseph): Because I love him.

Chris: What do you love about him?

Jenny (Joseph): He's very kind.

Chris: What else?

Jenny went on to list Joseph's numerous positive qualities and when prompted was able to give concrete examples of these qualities enacted. Then I asked:

Chris: What might be the very first small sign that Joseph is beginning to ignore your instructions?

Jenny (Joseph): He won't shut himself away. He tries to hide in his room when I'm angry.

Chris: What might he do instead?

Jenny (Joseph): He'll carry on with his routine.

Chris: What else will tell you that he is ignoring your instructions?

Jenny (Joseph): He'll keep taking his medication.

Chris: What difference do you think that will make?

Jenny (Joseph): He goes crazy when he stops his medication and that makes me even more angry.

Chris: What difference might it make to you if Joseph carries on with his routine and keeps taking his medication?

Jenny (Joseph): I won't have to worry about him so much.

Chris: What do you think will replace the worry?

Jenny (Joseph): Worry makes me angry so I won't get so angry.

Chris: What will replace the anger?

Jenny (Joseph): I'd be more calm.

Chris: What difference will that make?

Jenny (Joseph): We'd get along better.

I drew out a little more description of what "getting along better" might look like, then thanked Jenny and went back to a direct conversation with Joseph.

Chris: So, Joseph, what would be the first sign of this miracle happening? What would tell you that your life was beginning to move forward normally towards a job and possibly even marriage?

Joseph: I wouldn't lie in bed half the day.

Chris: What would you do instead?

The session now continued routinely without further asides to "Jenny." Joseph was able to describe many features of what, for him, would be a "normal" life. Later, on a zero to 10 scale where 10 represented a fully "normal" post-miracle life and zero meant no part of this life was present, Joseph rated himself at a 4. Our exploring what was already in place in Joseph's life led to a substantial historical base for the future he was seeking. He already worked one day a week in a charity bookshop, ate well, shopped and cooked for himself. He had several casual friends, one of whom he wanted to know better. As an afterthought, he added as he was leaving that he went to the cinema most weeks – with Jenny.

Joseph continued seeing me for a total of six sessions, timings decided by him, over the next three years. The last visit, after a year's gap, was to tell me how well he was doing. During this time, he made no further suicide attempts and had no hospital admissions. Donna, the psychiatrist, had stayed in occasional contact but was about to "discharge" him from her care. He had become a paid, part-time staff member at the bookshop, had a good social life, and had become a public speaker at events hosted by his "celebrity" family.

Joseph remained unmarried but continued to visit the cinema most weeks with Jenny.

Donna became a passionately Solution-Focused practitioner and referred many more of her clients, and we are still in touch.

Case #2: The White Cube: Death Defeated

The hospital was a crack in the beauty of its surrounding landscape of wild moorland. Victorian red brick with vestiges of factory gothic, two layers of tall windows stretching across its north-facing façade, and a chimney which both dwarfed and echoed the last of its sisters from the woolen mills. In a larger city it would already have been demolished for its land or turned into luxury apartments for young people oblivious of its tortured ghosts. But here, watching the perimeter of a declining northern town, the hospital continued to offer a bleak refuge for lost souls, many of whom, despite the odds, were being helped to find the first footholds back toward a better life.

I was there for a week, not as a patient; I was running a Solution-Focused Brief Therapy training for the mental-health staff. The transfer in the 1980s of all but the most intensive psychiatric treatments to community-based home-care services had, thankfully, seen the end of most nineteenth-century prison-like hospitals, many of which had been sold for their land. But this hospital, out in the wilds, was of little monetary value and was falling into disrepair. The training department for psychiatric services was located in an abandoned ward that had remained undecorated since it had been emptied more than two decades previously. Within this architecture of depression, it was not surprising to find the 36 course members in a somewhat low mood. Luckily, for teachers and learners, the business of learning how to be solution-focused is an enjoyable and energizing experience, so I was not unduly fazed by their initial lifelessness. By lunchtime, I was most definitely fazed; if anything, the group had become even more down-hearted, and I was beginning to doubt my own ability to last five days in such an atmosphere. As I was eating a dubious soup served with yesterday's bread, Miriam, the lead psychiatrist who had arranged the training, sat down and explained the gloom.

They were expecting a death. Rosa, a suicidal young woman, had been admitted over the weekend and was being detained against her will, so she could be force-fed. Though only 19 she was well known to the hospital. From the age of 12 she had been struggling against a compulsion to starve herself to death and was now close to losing the struggle. Being familiar with the system, she had come prepared, this time, with a lethal overdose sewn into her clothing. Only the vigilance of a nursing assistant had saved her, but pumping out her stomach had left her very weak. The staff could either risk killing her by force-feeding or let her die from starvation. This was not the first time that I had encountered desperate patients being protected from self-harm on locked wards, nor was it the first time I had offered to meet with the client. Putting the evidence, limited as it was, that there was an 80% chance of Solution-Focused Brief Therapy leading to some lasting improvements in the client's life (Shennan & Iveson, 2011), I asked Miriam if she would like me to see Rosa that evening after the course. Already on the horns of a dilemma and thinking that it couldn't make things any worse, Miriam put the offer to Rosa and Rosa accepted.

At five o'clock, when the course finished for the day, Miriam and I crossed the hillside to the hospital's part-functioning west wing and began the long walk through a corridor flanked by abandoned rooms and almost palpably abandoned hope. The final door, opened by a key that might have come from a medieval dungeon, led us into the secure ward.

It was all but empty, though unlike the rest of the hospital it had received a recent coat of white paint that served to highlight even more the wire caging that guarded the windows, television, and security cameras. A scattering of beanbags provided the only furnishing for Rosa, who stood, so thin, almost transparent, beside one of the tall Gothic windows that had at one time given this building a coating of elegance.

As the three of us, an Asian Muslim psychiatrist, a (non-believing) Christian English-Irish-Scottish brief therapist and a Jewish client, settled ourselves on our beanbags, I drove away my vanity-fueled fear of looking foolish when the time came to stand up and my arthritic limbs failed to straighten. Rosa, pale-skinned, large-eyed and impassive, sat upright on her cushion. She knew she was close to death.

Whatever had brought Rosa to this so-sad state would have been explored, documented, hypothesized about, diagnosed, and treated – all to no effect so far. She had slipped through the various theories and treatment modalities and, despite the vast reaches of the medical model, she was doomed. So, why had she agreed to see me, a therapist? There must have been a good reason. There always is.

In the early days of Solution-Focused Brief Therapy there had been a three-part classification of motivation – "customer, complainant, and visitor" (de Shazer, 1985, 1988). BRIEF's first outcome study (Iveson, 1991) showed these classifications to have no predictive value, at least as far as our assessment skills went. The supposedly unmotivated clients did as well as those deemed to be highly motivated. From our point of view, we had to act on this finding and so chose to experiment by treating all clients as if they were motivated. Almost 30 years later we have discovered no evidence from our own practice to abandon this position. When we ask our opening question, "What are your best hopes from our talking together?" we expect to arrive at an answer that we and the client can work toward. The answer may not always come easily but it does not occur to us it won't come – it is part of our job. What is impossible to know is whether the client arrives with "motivation" or that "motivation" is constructed through the conversation – but in order to make such a construction, the therapist must act as if it is true, so the distinction is clinically irrelevant. Therefore, we work on the assumption that all clients have a "good reason" for being and remaining in a conversation with a therapist. This "good reason" could be that they want to keep their freedom or their children, it could be because they want to achieve something that is proving hard to reach, it could be because they still have, somewhere, the last glimmer of hope that a better life is possible. Our job is to discover that "good reason" and make it the starting point for a useful collaboration.

Once we realized that "motivation" was a constructive process and part of the therapeutic task, we have always worked with "motivated" clients, and in 25 years of running a free clinic for people in extreme difficulty, we have never turned a client away. If they come through the door, even when they are mandated, we see them as motivated and see our job as discovering what they are motivated for. Once we know that we can ask our "miracle questions" to open up descriptions of preferred futures, and we can use scales to chart the histories of those futures. That is all that is necessary for an effective therapy averaging three sessions (Gingerich & Peterson, 2013; Shennan & Iveson, 2011).

All this was forgotten in the intensity of the first seconds of our meeting; Miriam had all but disappeared, it was just me and Rosa who returned my interest with a stare empty of life. To my opening question, "What are your best hopes from our talking together?," she answered with such flatness and despair it could have extinguished the sun: "I don't do hope."

Remembering it now, I can still feel a shiver at the back of my neck as, for a moment, a pit began to open before me. What hubris had brought me here? What had led me to imagine that I had anything to offer this young woman so close to her death, so determined to die? As these thoughts threatened to drag me down into Rosa's pit of hopelessness, they were suddenly replaced by something close to joy. What an extraordinary privilege it was to be allowed to sit on the very cliff edge of another person's death and invite her back to life. That was all I had to do. I didn't have to understand her or understand what was driving her to this dreadful place. I didn't have to "cure" her or fix her or make her life somehow right. All I had to do was ask another question, a question that contained an invitation to life.

Chris: If you did? If you did do hope?

Rosa: (With the same flat tone) I...don't...do...hope.

I will always owe to Rosa the confidence these two answers gave to my future work. Confidence in the realization that all I ever have to do is ask the next question, and as each question is answered, there is a chance that the next answer will include an acceptance of my invitation to take a small step toward life, toward a more livable future. As Rosa reiterated her refusal to hope, I saw, with the clarity of a vision, the task before me. In my mind we had entered a "white cube," a room devoid of all features and not only had the door closed behind us, it had been erased forever. The only way out of this cube-like room was through a second door known only to Rosa. My job was to ask the questions that would bring Rosa to a discovery of this knowledge only she possessed: the whereabouts of the second door – the door to life. When she found it, we could both leave and go our separate ways. Since my meeting with the extraordinary Rosa, this "vision" has supported my journeys with many people close to preferring death instead of their almost unlivable lives and given me the hopefulness that awakens the next question, and the next.

Still in search of Rosa's "good reason" for seeing me, the conversation progressed to the third question.

Chris: How come you agreed to see me?

Rosa: It's something to do.

Chris: Is it? Seeing a counselor? Most people in here would run a mile before seeing someone like me!

Rosa: That's true!

Chris: So how come you agreed?

Rosa: You don't know how bad it is in here!

Chris: Don't you like it?

Rosa: What do you think?

Chris: I don't know, but I bet there are people here that like it so much they can't be persuaded to leave.

Rosa: (with the first sign of animation) Well, I'm not one of them!

Chris: So, you want to leave?

Rosa: (forcefully) Yes, I do!

Then I felt the psychiatrist shift her position, and a new tension entered the room. She and Rosa knew where this was going, to leave in a coffin, and both assumed that I didn't.

Chris: So, if our meeting in some way helps you leave here, that means it will have been useful?

Rosa: Maybe

Chris: I mean leave here in a way that is right for you?

Rosa: (with renewed animation) Yes!

Miriam was now becoming quite agitated and was likely at any moment to call a halt, to stop me, apparently, working with Rosa toward her death since Rosa had told the hospital staff earlier that she intended to leave the hospital in a coffin.

I have never wanted to kill myself, but I could imagine that if I did, I would not regard seeing a counselor as the right route for such a venture, and neither can I imagine amusing myself with idle conversation. Consequently, I assumed that Rosa, at some level, possibly not even obvious to herself, had not entirely given up. It was this Rosa I was looking for, the Rosa with a "good reason," but with very little time before the psychiatrist called a halt to what she was beginning to believe was a misguided and possibly dangerous conversation.

Chris: So, let's imagine that tonight, while you are asleep, a miracle happens; it doesn't get you out of here, but what it does do is set off the process which will enable you to leave this hospital ... (*Miriam was now like a kettle about to blow its lid and I hoped that what I said next, though vital to the invitation, would shock her into a silence just long enough for me to finish my question) ...* leave this hospital in a way that is absolutely right for you *... (Now Rosa was almost aglow with anticipation of the death she had been working toward for so many years) ...* absolutely right for you – and right for the hospital. What will be the first thing that you notice that tells you that a miracle has happened?

As "right for the hospital" was spoken, Miriam slumped with relief and the light went out of Rosa's eyes. There was a pause as we made room for her answer, and then she let out a long sigh. It was a sigh that I have heard many times since, and though it carries with it a sadness, it seemed to mark the start of a decision to give life another chance, hard work though that would be. Following the sigh, Rosa said:

Rosa: I suppose I wouldn't feel so bad when I woke up.

Chris: How would you feel instead?

Rosa: I wouldn't be happy.

Chris: So how do you think you would feel after this miracle, even if you weren't actually feeling happy?

Rosa: I don't know, maybe a sense of just getting on with it.

Chris: What time would that be?

Rosa: Too early! When they start clanking around and changing shifts.

Chris: Who might be the first to notice at that early time that you had woken up ready to "get on with it"?

Rosa: Probably Angela. She's one of the ward sisters and she's on this week.

Chris: What do you think Angela might notice that gives her the first hint that this miracle has happened and you have decided to "get on with it"?

Rosa: (laughing) I'll say "Good morning" to her.

Chris: Will she be surprised or does that happen anyway?

Rosa: She'll definitely be surprised – I don't talk to anyone at that time!

Chris: How do you think she'll respond?

Rosa: She'll probably want to hug me!

Chris: Would you like that?

Rosa: (looking at her body) As long as she didn't snap me in half!

Chris: What would Angela notice about your response to her hug that fitted with you deciding to "get on with it"?

Rosa: I'd probably tell her she didn't have to worry, not this time anyway.

Chris: How might she respond to that?

Rosa: Knowing Angela, she'd probably cry – we'd both probably cry!

Chris: What might be the next small sign that this miracle had happened?

The chain of questions had begun. Rosa described what she, other patients, and staff members would notice the following morning as she began her long and difficult journey back to a life worth living. Later in the session, when describing what was keeping her just above zero on a 10-point scale where ten represented the life after the miracle that she had been describing for most of the session, Rosa reluctantly admitted that to have lived through what she had lived through had required many great strengths, and that these strengths just might serve her well in the challenges ahead.

In cases such as Rosa's my first task is to establish a legitimate outcome. Rosa's ostensible "hope" was for death, but she would be perfectly cognizant of the restrictions on my endeavors. For most of us, helping a client commit suicide would be unethical, and Rosa would not have expected me to go down this path. Instead, I offered her a path which fitted her spoken wish to leave hospital "in a way that was right" for her, and added the legitimate safeguarding limitation on the available routes. It would be the same with other mandated clients: caring for your children in a way that is absolutely right for you and also right for the authorities; staying out of jail in a way that is absolutely right for you and right for the court.

Structurally, the session was a "textbook case": about five minutes to establish a desired outcome, 30 or so minutes describing the fine detail of a realistic tomorrow, and around 15 minutes using a scale to uncover the history of the client's preferred future. In place of finishing by giving Rosa compliments or commendations, I asked Miriam to tell me what she knew about Rosa that gave Miriam hope that Rosa would somehow win through to a better life. Miriam had plenty to say, much of it a pleasant surprise to Rosa.

The following morning Miriam arrived late for the course. She had been to see Rosa, who she found, for the first time, in the dining room. She had declined breakfast ("I never eat breakfast!") but was drinking a cup of tea. To Miriam and the entire group this was indeed a miracle. For several years, while Miriam was in charge, I returned every year to train all the new staff in Solution-Focused Brief Therapy. Which meant that I saw Rosa one more time.

It was the following year and the same grim surroundings were lit up by a bunch of enthusiastic mental-health professionals eager to learn about Solution-Focused Brief Therapy. Miriam came by not just to say hello but to ask if I would see Rosa again as she was back in hospital. My initial disappointment was lifted when Miriam said it was a "breakthrough." For the first time ever, Rosa had asked to be admitted. A new yearning toward death had appeared but this time she was planning to fight it. The inpatient treatment had started well but, in Miriam's words, had gone "pear-shaped" and they were fast sinking back into old patterns. Once again, I met with Rosa, this time in the less dwarfing environs of Miriam's office. She was ready for my questions. She had no hope at all, let alone any "best hopes," and for 45 minutes we played a "cat-and-mouse" game around this question revolving around the inconsistency of just wanting to die and agreeing to see a very persistent therapist. After those 45 minutes I must have hit upon the right question because she suddenly admitted that there were things she needed to do before dying. This opened the way for an agreement:

Chris: So, if our talk today led you to be able to live with less pain and stress for the time that you are alive, would that mean it had been useful?

Rosa: I suppose so.

Chris: So, let's imagine that you wake up tomorrow feeling less pain, less stress – what would you notice instead?

After a few minutes of an almost exact repeat of last year's dialogue, Rosa said: "Okay, okay!" and turning to Miriam, said, "He doesn't take any nonsense, does he!"

Eight years later Miriam moved on and I was swept away by a new broom. Rosa was still "on the books" but just for six-monthly reviews. She was also married with two children.

Conclusion: "It's the Questions, Isn't It?"

It can be argued that Solution-Focused Brief Therapy has only three questions:

- *What are your best hopes from our work together?*
- *How will your life be different if these hopes are realized?*
- *What are you already doing or have done in the past that might help bring these hopes to fruition?*

Every question we ask is a variation of these. Nothing else is necessary. The content, the words that make a difference to the clients' lives, all come from the clients. This knowledge might not ever be tapped without the questions and, no doubt, some of it is co-constructed by the question-answer process, but none of the content can be owned by the therapist. Each time a therapist asks a question a client has never been asked before, the answer is likely to be something the client has never heard before – this is the client's knowledge. The therapist's job is to find versions of the three questions that lead the client to say those words that open up new meanings, new possibilities, a new life for the client. In those seemingly hopeless cases where the therapist feels at the very edge of his or her skills, it might also be claimed that the questions have an element of creativity.

At the end of a single session that had a transformative effect – with Carrie, another client (Iveson et al., 2014) – the following brief dialogue said it all:

Carrie: It's the questions, isn't it?

Chris: I'm not so sure about that – I think it's more likely to be the answers.

Carrie: I know that, but I wouldn't have had those answers without the questions.

References

de Shazer, S. (1985). *Keys to solution in brief therapy.* New York: Norton.

de Shazer, S. (1988). *Clues: Investigating solutions in brief therapy.* New York: Norton.

Gingerich, W. J., & Peterson, L. T. (2013). Effectiveness of solution-focused brief therapy: A systematic qualitative review of controlled outcome studies. *Research in Social Work Practice, 23*(3), 266–283.

Iveson, C., George, E., & Ratner, H. (2014). Love is all around: A single session solution-focused therapy. In M.F. Hoyt, & M. Talmon (Eds.). *Capturing the moment: Single session therapy and walk-in services* (pp. 325–348). Bethel, CT: Crown House.

Iveson, D. (1991). *Outcomes in solution focused brief therapy.* Unpublished Masters Dissertation. Birkbeck College. University of London.

Ratner, H., George, E., & Iveson, C. (2012). *Solution focused brief therapy: 100 key points and techniques.* London: Routledge.

Shennan, G., & Iveson, C. (2011). From solution to description: Practice and research in tandem. In C. Franklin, T.S. Trepper, W.J. Gingerich, & E.E. McCollum (Eds.). *Solution-focused brief therapy: A handbook of evidence-based practice* (pp. 281–298). New York: Oxford University Press.

Tomm, K., Hoyt, M.F., & Madigan, S.P. (1998). Honoring our internalized others and the ethics of caring: A conversation with Karl Tomm. In M.F. Hoyt (Ed.). *Handbook of constructive therapies: Innovative approaches from leading practitioners* (pp. 198–218). San Francisco: Jossey-Bass.

CHAPTER 13

120 Centimeters from Sainthood

Hillary Keeney and Bradford Keeney

The following session was conducted in front of an audience during a ten-day seminar in Budapest, Hungary in 2014, sponsored by Dr. Dezsoe Birkas, Director of the Budapest Institute for Systemic Brief Therapy. Each day we conducted several live demonstration interviews with clients who brought a wide range of presenting issues, including behavioral problems, presumed psychiatric disorders, marital and relationship crises, family conflict, grief, and physical illness. The purpose of the seminar was to demonstrate how more creative choices of action arise when practitioners break free from the limitations of any form of habituated therapy protocol, diagnostic classification scheme, and advocated theoretical orientation and instead become organized by building a vaster, more resourceful existential "room" or "frame" for the client's life. We have previously described this approach as *improvisational therapy* (Keeney, 1991), *creative therapy* (Keeney, 2009), and *circular therapeutics* (H. Keeney & B. Keeney, 2012). Regardless of the name used, our orientation remains focused on a non-psychological approach that regards each session's structure as a three-act play that improvisationally unfolds from an entrenched beginning, to a transformational middle, and finally to an expanded ending where more possibilities and greater creative energy are found.

In the transcription that follows we limit our commentary to tracking the movement from impoverished, constricted frames to resourceful, expanded frames (H. Keeney, B. Keeney, & Chenail, 2015) – what we sometimes simply refer to as going from a "small room" to a "big room." Clients come seeking change – movement from their current impoverished situation to one that is more resourceful, interesting, expansive, positive, and full of life. The specific description, interpretation, or understanding of the presenting problem, the sought solution, or the desired destination is less important than the movement itself. In fact, creative improvisation in therapy is hampered by too much emphasis on the presumption that practitioners must first understand or accurately interpret what is going on in a client's life (whether the hermeneutics of problems, solutions, narratives, politics, or systemic contexts) before acting to introduce any creative difference that leads to transformation. Rather than join clients in perpetuating the same way of first knowing and then subsequently acting in relationship to their life circumstance, we immediately hunt for any opportunity to make an exit toward new territory without preconceived notions of how we will get there and what will arise along the way. Creative change lies outside the box of both the practitioner's and client's knowing, and that fertile ground is only reached by surrendering to the greater mind and dance of interaction that can deliver unexpected bigger surprises that may include a new mission for a man's life.

Session Transcription with Commentary

"József" is a Hungarian man in his mid-thirties who had been seeing a therapist specializing in treating psychosomatic illness. József was invited by his therapist, Dr. Birkas, to have one session with us in front of the seminar audience. Names and identifying details have been altered to protect the client's privacy. Permission was obtained from the client to record and publish the transcription of this session and a professional translator was present during the session to offer Hungarian-English translation. József did not attend the seminar nor did he witness any other demonstration interviews. This session was the first time we met József and we had no knowledge of his situation or therapeutic history prior to the session. After exchanging initial greetings, József sits down and describes his condition.

József: I've had a skin illness for ten years. It is like a painful rash with wounds. Dermatologists say that it is incurable. It causes a lot of inconveniences in my life. I cannot move properly, there is a lot of pain, and it also smells because it bleeds. I don't leave home very much because of it. The rash is on six different parts of my body. I'm on government assistance because I cannot work.

Brad: Has it always been on six different parts of your body?

Brad underscores what stood out as unique about József's description of his condition: the rash is on *six different parts* of his body. The mention of this number of body parts is the description that encourages the most creative exploration. Though we do not yet know where a line of questioning about the "six different parts" will lead, we choose to emphasize or re-indicate this interesting fact rather than pursue a more elaborated definition and reification of József's suffering.

József: No, first it was under the left underarm. In the beginning it was one blister, and the doctors said it was acne.

Hillary: It went from being on one part of you to six parts of you?

József: First it was on the left underarm, then the blister broke, and then it spread to the right underarm and it kept spreading.

Brad: [Begins pointing to different parts of József's body] Okay, so it's here, here, here...

József: Yes, under both underarms, on the stomach, in the groin, on my chest, and on my bottom.

Brad: [Starts counting while pointing to the different parts of the body he is naming] So one, two, three, four, five, six. Is the condition going to stop at six places?

József: Now there are a lot of wounds on six places. Probably yes, the number of places will stop, but the number of wounds in those six places will increase.

As we explore the theme of "six different parts," including whether the rash began on one part of the body and spread, as well as drawing attention to the specific parts of József's body where it is located, the conversation builds a frame or context that underscores what is unique about the rash, dissociating it from any standardized definition of the presumed disease. We find that the rash is not only on six particular parts of the body, it is also able to *change* – move to different locations. Inside this frame a question pops into Brad's mind that takes the conversation in a new direction:

Brad: It's a strange thing to think, but what if you had the wounds on the palms of your hands and on the bottoms of your feet, and around your head? If that were the case, you would have thousands of people coming to touch you.

József: [Chuckles] I think the wounds are so ugly that people wouldn't want to touch me.

Brad: But if your wounds were on those places – hands, feet, and head – it would be called stigmata. It's a strange thought, isn't it? It would be strange if you woke up one morning and the wounds were here, on the palms of your hands. [Brad points to József's palms]

József: [József nods and smiles] All the Catholics would come and stroke me.

Here an entirely new consideration is offered: If the rash moved to the hands, feet, and head it would transform into a revered mystical and religiously important sign (a "stigmata"), rather than a despised illness. Brad's introduction of this new frame within a larger context opens a door to the first major movement forward in the session. The rash, formerly regarded only as an illness that negatively impacts József's life, is now under consideration as a special mystery that may even bring József public recognition and acclaim. It's notable that József quickly imagines that if his rash moved locations and became stigmata that he would be publicly adored ("All the Catholics would come and stroke me.")

Brad: It's true! Let's see here. *[Brad studies József's arm, pointing first to his underarm where the wounds currently are, and then tracing his finger down to József's palm]* So you are this far from being a saint. *[József and the audience laugh]*

József: 120 centimeters.

Hillary: Wow, you know the distance between your shoulder and your hand! How do you know this?

József: Because before my illness I played professional water polo, and the length of the arm is very important.

Brad: 120 centimeters. That's quite a thought! Right now that's what I would name your case. If I were going to write up some notes about you in a case file, I would title your case "120 Centimeters from Sainthood," and that would be true. Because if your condition walked 120 centimeters down the length of your arm from here *[points to József's underarm]* to here *[points to his palm]*, then thousands, maybe a million Catholics and Protestants – everyone actually – would come to touch you.

József: Would that be good?

Hillary: I don't know. It would certainly be an interesting change for you. You might have to hide.

Brad: Yes, and wouldn't that be something. Because in a way you've been dress rehearsing for how to hide. You've become an expert on hiding. Maybe you've been getting ready for this.

The conversation has moved, along with the rash, inside the new frame that József's somatic situation may be an indication that he is only "120 centimeters from sainthood." This frame allows us to revisit and challenge what was previously only a singularly negative impact of the rash – being confined to his house and not working. With the frame change, the rash brings something potentially beneficial, a "dress rehearsal" for a possible future display of adoration that would require József to hide from public devotion. Additional discussion of the suffering brought by his rash further bolsters the theme that he is 120 centimeters from sainthood and has been preparing for this unexpected, and even historic, dramatically important role.

Brad: It would be interesting if you drew a little road – just in your imagination – from your underarm down to your palm, with a little sign and arrow that points the way toward your palm.

Hillary: In fact you can do it right now – just hold your arm out and draw a line all the way to your palm. *[József lifts his right arm forward, palm facing up, and takes his other hand and draws an imaginary line from his underarm all the way down to his palm]*

Brad: That's right. And put a little arrow here, pointing toward your palm. Then, when it's time and when you're ready, you can say to your wounds: "You can now travel 120 centimeters to my palm." *[József turns his face toward his underarm and speaks these words quietly to his wounds]*

Brad: Now, because you said those words and drew that road, the deepest part of your mind has heard that this is a possibility. It's possible that now you may have a dream in the night or in the day, a fantasy or a very vivid dream, that this wound – step by step – marches down the highway 120 steps, 120 centimeters, and comes home. If you had that dream, you would begin to wonder: "Maybe what has happened to me is more than what doctors can see. There is something that is a mystery about me and my life, and my wounds, and my being 120 steps, 120 centimeters, away from sainthood." Now I'm going to tell you a very big secret: your life would be a nightmare if you received the stigmata, because thousands of people would be coming to see you and driving you crazy. Hundreds of thousands of people would come to you. It would be a nightmare. You would get on your knees and pray, "Please Lord, tell my stigmata to walk 120 centimeters back to be hidden under my arm." So the question is, is it a gift that you received a wound that is hidden? Or can you, your heart, and your soul fulfill this bigger mystery of your life in ways that touch people's lives and touch their hearts? Can you fulfill this mystery without fear, knowing that the people will regard you as someone who can give them everything?

As the mystery of József's rash is further taken to indicate that he is just "120 centimeters from sainthood," József is invited to reconsider whether his former reality, that of a man who suffers greatly from a bad rash, might actually be less problematic than being a saint. Saints, after all, are not only respected and exalted but are known for their willingness to undergo great suffering and self-sacrifice in order to live a life of piety and generosity for the sake of others. Brad takes the two primary frames of the session, "Man who suffers from a rash" and "120 centimeters from sainthood," and places them side by side for József to compare. The exciting new possibility that his life is marked by spiritual mystery is tempered by the fact that it would also mean he would have to step into a bigger role in the world and likely face even more suffering, though his rash would then be a resource and badge of honor rather than a disease that carries the mark of shame. This consideration invites József to wonder whether his current situation, having his wounds hidden, might actually be preferable or even a gift that gets him off the hook from sainthood.

Hillary: Our guess is that you have a soft heart.

József: I've never thought about it.

Brad: Our guess is that you are soft, and that if somebody needs help, you want to help them.

József: Yes. Mostly I am this way with my family.

Brad: Yes, and if these wounds were here on your palm, you would have a hard time saying no to people who need help.

József: [Nods] Yes. Do you think it is easier this way, with the wounds here? [He points under his arm]

Brad: Oh yes, it is much easier to have the wounds here [points to József's underarm] than here [points to József's palm]. Are you a religious man?

József: No.

Brad: Then you're very lucky that the wounds are hidden under your arm. If they were on your palm, you would have to be very religious. [Brad smiles and József and the audience laugh] You are 120 centimeters away from being totally religious, from being worshipped. But because you are 120 centimeters away, you are closer than other people who have no wounds like yours. It's just an interesting thing to consider. It brings interesting possibilities to your life. Are you aware that there are doctors who believe that what happens to the skin – where a wound is located and how far it is away from other parts of the body – is a communication? Do you know this?

József: Yes.

Brad: Doctors will often give an interpretation based on what they see on the skin, just as someone could look at the way you sit and the way you walk and say that these say something about you. Some would say these things on your skin say something about you. All I know is that your wound is 120 centimeters from your palm. Have you ever considered being religious for one hour?

József: No. I'm baptized and I'm a member of the Reformed Church, but I'm not a believer.

Brad: It's very interesting – this 120 centimeters. 120 centimeters, 120 steps, maybe 120 minutes. That's two hours. Maybe you need a two-hour experiment in saying "thank you" to the universe. Would that work for you – saying thank you to the universe? You could say, "Thank you for not putting the wound on my hand, but instead putting it here under my arm, because otherwise everyone would think that I'm a believer." Because some of the saints – those who believed the most and prayed the most – received the wound here. [Brad points to József's palm] Maybe for 120 minutes you could say "thank you" that your wound is not on your palm. Or maybe you could say "thank you" 120 times. Then you could write down the number 120 on your palm – each palm. Throughout each day, think of this number. When you wake up in the morning, say "120." When you go to sleep, say "120." Put 120 in your life in many, many ways, without knowing why. Just do it to honor the fact that the road from here to here is one 120 centimeters away. *[Brad traces his finger from József's underarm down to his palm]* You might live an additional 120 more years because you say the number 120 so often. You might change 120 people's lives during your lifetime. I don't know how 120 will show up for you in other ways in your life.

After inviting József to reconsider his current situation as fortunate when contrasted with the possibility that he may have to dedicate his life to serving the multitudes, we return fully to the heart of the theme of his being just 120 centimeters from sainthood. After establishing that József already has the "soft heart" required for a saintlier role in the world, the conversation turns to exploring all the ways József can experiment with honoring this mystery in his daily life without having to suddenly become "religious" or a saint. The mystery itself is contained in the distance – 120 centimeters or steps – between his current situation and an imagined future reality. Several prescriptions are mentioned for creative action that invite József to further celebrate and elaborate the mystery of "120" and allow it to permeate his thoughts and actions.

Brad: *[Brad leans forward and takes hold of József's hand. He gets a vibration in his voice and speaks slowly]* I do know that every time you catch yourself thinking "Why this? Why that?," if instead you start thinking about 120, then *[BAM! Brad claps his hands once very loudly]* something will wake up, deep inside of you. *[József begins to weep]* 120 centimeters, 120 songs, 120 children, 120 fathers, 120 days, and 120 nights. I think you should flood your life with the number 120, for 120 days. Get a calendar. Each day mark one day of "120," then the second day of "120." Do it because you are 120 centimeters away from sainthood. You received the hood that covers the wounds. *[A church bell is heard ringing outside the window]* And now the bell rings! Every time you hear the church bell ring, say "120." From time to time and for no reason at all, just say "120" out loud. *[The church bell continues to ring]* The bell is ringing for the next saint. Saint 120. We are making that number a saint, and you have a relationship with that number. *[Brad whispers]* There's nothing else we should say, other than the next time we see you, we'll say "Hello, Saint 120." Thank you.

József: *[Both weeping and smiling widely, begins nodding]*. Thank you! *[Brad, Hillary, and József stand and embrace. The audience claps.]*

In the final moments of the session, Brad further amplified the emotion and energy that had grown in the conversation as it moved toward exploring the mystery that József's condition, previously assumed to be strictly problematic, might actually be a hidden solution to what could have been or could become a major social challenge for him: being regarded as a saint rather than someone in a need of healing. As Brad underscored this bigger view that was nearer than anyone thought (only 120 centimeters away), he did so with an increasingly loud voice that finally broke into a tremble with a slower and a more declaratory manner of speech. He finally clapped his hand loudly as if hitting a peak level to make an exclamatory punctuation. It resulted in József weeping as he was emotionally touched by feeling near more mystery in his life.

120 Centimeters from Change

Several weeks after this session, it occurred to us that it would be highly unusual for a man's arm to measure 120 centimeters from shoulder to palm. Curious about this, our colleague and József's therapist, Dr. Birkas, asked József about this number. József replied that it wasn't until after the session that he too realized this was not his actual measurement, and he was filled with even more of a sense of mystery about it, wondering why this number, 120 centimeters, arose with such certainty for him. József found out an interesting fact that links this measurement to the Church of Nativity in Bethlehem. It is the only church in the Holy Land that has survived since the early Christian period and it has a small entrance door that some have measured as 120 centimeters high. It is called "The Door of Humility" and it symbolizes the equality of all people before God.

Three months after the seminar his therapist and physician told us that after our session József found it unexplainably difficult to touch his skin when it itched or was irritated – he mentioned that something held him back from a previous automatic habit. We also learned that a month later, while József was taking a bath, he panicked because he suddenly felt paralyzed and could not move. Having previously been a professional water polo player, this was truly a shock for him to not be able to move while in the water. After his initial panic, however, József became curious whether that episode of paralysis was simply another mysterious change in his symptoms. As the habits that formerly contributed to perpetuating his irritated skin were interrupted for reasons he did not understand, József was able to move on with his life without the flare-ups he had previously experienced. Two years later József attended a public musical presentation we performed in Budapest on global healing traditions. Dr. Birkas told us that during the reception after the event, József announced to several of the attendees, "The Keeneys taught me it can be useful to do the opposite of whatever your habits usually want you to do."

József did not identify himself as a religious man, but yet the mystery of his skin condition and the conversation it inspired invite all of us to consider that there may be more to every life situation than what initially meets the eye. No matter what the specific nature of the suffering a client brings, make it your mission to get every session moving in a bigger direction where there is more room for mystery. Consider following József's tracks and welcome both you and your client doing the opposite of your habituated routines. Be more ready and willing to not know what you will say or do in a session before the interaction begins. Listen for the intuitive whisper of an improbable theme and pay more attention to the sensory experience of unexplainable irregularities from numbers to symbols, sounds, and movements. With these more mysterious exceptionalities in hand, build up a context that inverts, reverses, spins, alters, and changes all who participate within (Keeney & Keeney, 2013).

In the case of József, the first important crossroads of the session was presented in his opening remarks. Had we chosen to invite elaboration of the impoverishing effects József's skin condition had on his life it would have kept the session residing inside the theme of the presenting pathology, delaying or even blocking entirely the advancement of the session somewhere different, an existential territory bursting with more surprise. Instead, we immediately picked up on the one piece of József's initial communication that held the most possibility for a new kind of exploration: the rash travels around "six different parts" of his body. This enabled us to find a pathway to a more enriched and resourceful way of relating to his presenting communication, through both metaphor and embodied action.

Because every client and session bring different circumstances, it isn't possible to anticipate what will be observed, served, heard, or contextually turned. Rather than know what should generally be said or unsaid, done or left undone, pay more attention to discerning the unexpected and then build up a space where the uncommon, unique, unusual, and creative are in full force, providing a resourceful source of change.

We invite you to be inspired by this Hungarian swimmer who resisted the habitual itch, resulting in more interest in mystery than former misery. You, too, are no more than "120 centimeters" from changing how you will conduct your next session. How far is your body, this very moment, from the "120" marked on this page? You also can benefit from cutting yourself a length of string that is 120 centimeters long, or hanging a picture of the number 120 on your wall, or even from time to time, writing the number 120 on your palm. Do this and remember how close you always are to the bigger mystery that surrounds every mundane, habituated frame offered in a session.

Søren Kierkegaard believed that no one is far away from sainthood, including rascals and scoundrels: "God creates out of nothing, wonderful, you say: yes, to be sure, but he does what is still more wonderful: he makes saints out of sinners" (Kierkegaard, 2003, p. 59). Practitioners are also called to help clients create something extraordinary out of what may seem like "nothing" – a seemingly hopeless situation. Every session is an opportunity to uncover the mystery of the greater whole of life that remains hidden when held inside impoverished frames and shrunken contexts. If you have already worked with more than 120 clients, or experienced at least 120 sessions, or have more than

120 seconds before your next session, then go ahead and improvise and utilize whatever measured distance helps you and your client traverse the nearest path to a bigger life.

References

Keeney, B. P. (1991). *Improvisational therapy: A practical guide for creative clinical strategies*. New York: Guilford Press.

Keeney, B. P. (2009). *The creative therapist: The art of awakening a session*. New York: Routledge.

Keeney, H. & Keeney, B. (2012). *Circular therapeutics: Giving therapy a healing heart*. Phoenix, AZ: Zeig, Tucker & Theisen.

Keeney, H. & Keeney, B. (2013). *Creative therapeutic technique: Skills for the art of bringing forth change*, Phoenix, AZ: Zeig, Tucker & Theisen.

Keeney, H., Keeney, B., & Chenail, R. (2015). *Recursive frame analysis: A qualitative research method for mapping change-oriented discourse*. Fort Lauderdale, FL: The Qualitative Report Books.

Kierkegaard, S. (2003). *The soul of Kierkegaard: Selections from his journal* (A. Dru, Ed.). Mineola, NY: Dover Publications.

CHAPTER 14

Random Effects of Ambiguity Along the Pathway Toward Health

David V. Keith

The therapeutic work described in this chapter is grounded in Symbolic Experiential Family Therapy, a therapeutic pattern outside the family therapy mainstream (wherever that may be). If conventional family therapy is concert music, Symbolic Experiential Therapy would be folk music with jazz chording. It looks simple on the surface but the simplicity disappears when you try to play it.

I am going to describe two novel clinical experiences that led to therapeutic change. Both were spontaneous comments grounded in what I call "poetic knowing." Poetic knowing infers a different kind of knowing from applied science or the more purposeful knowing that goes with psychoeducation. Symbolic Experiential Therapy is an atheoretical way of working. It is grounded not in a theory, but rather it is based on clinical experience, better, the accumulation of clinical experience. Carl Whitaker, my mentor and ultimately good friend, said long ago, "I have a theory that theories are destructive – and I *know* intuition is destructive. Isn't it sad? And no excuses will be accepted" (Whitaker, 1976/1982, p. 317).

The conceptual basis is a bit like a stew: it has many ingredients that have cooked together so long that it is hard to discern the different components. The ingredients include slices of eco-systemic theory concepts, several heaping tablespoons of Winnicott, a quarter cup of psychoanalytic theoretical vermouth, hypnotherapy, existential philosophy, dialectical thinking, Umberto Eco, theater of the absurd, Zen, play therapy, James Joyce, experiential therapy with psychotic patients, and more recently readings from semioticians, just to mention some of the more prominent components. The therapists who work with me tend to be people who read, and talk about what they read. Our understanding of how to operationalize this kind of thinking in the clinic has emerged gradually over years of clinical practice, teaching, writing and conversation with like-minded colleagues. It continues to evolve (Keith & Kaye, 2001).

When I report on my clinical experiences some jump to the conclusion that "anything goes." That is never true. You are responsible for what you do and what you say in clinical work and "no excuses are accepted." I am going to describe two experiences that fit the *"You Said What?"* context of this book. And while both examples come out of the poetics of random spontaneity, what was said was said by an experienced and responsible version of the author.

Please keep in mind: this kind of psychotherapy is an art. And "Art is a habit of intellect developed with practice over time that empowers the artist to make the work right and protects him … from deviating from what is good for the work. It unites what he is with what his material is. It leads him to seek his own depths. Its purpose is not self-enhancement, his having fun or feeling good about himself. These are byproducts…" (hooks, 1995, p. vi).

A fundamental principle of Symbolic Experiential Therapy is that the dynamics of psychotherapy are in the personhood of the therapist. It might be useful to know a little about this author/therapist. I am a psychiatrist. But I am a family-systems psychiatrist. The family-systems mindset is different from conventional modern psychiatry. I am a medication minimalist (see Prosky & Keith, 2003). I started out in internal medicine and moved to psychiatry because I was most interested in perplexingly ambiguous patients, people with psychosomatic disorders and with serious disruptions like psychosis, or treatment-resistant depression.

One of the first steps in my becoming a psychotherapist was the emergence of a depathologized view of psychosis. I gradually became aware of my belief that psychosis is a vehicle not a destiny. Psychosis is an effort to get somewhere, unless it is arrested and it ends up nowhere. Working with these more difficult situations, whether problems of the body, of the emotions, or of the relational systems requires careful listening, attention to language and how it is used. Most particularly it means tuning into metaphorical reality, letting words and phrases mean more than what is explicitly intended. A key to relating to psychotic people is being attuned to metaphorical reality. In both of the clinical situations described here, I was attuned to metaphorical reality.

Further, I believe that all we view as psychopathology is grounded in interpersonal experience. If pathology emerges from interpersonal experience, it can be disrupted or integrated with interpersonal experience. Of course, neither of the patients described here would be diagnosed as psychotic, but psychosis exists at one end of a continuum in how language is used. Following my compadre Whitaker, I think we are all "schizophrenic."

The Language of Psychotherapy

For the sake of simplicity and brevity, there are two kinds of language: (1) practical (or constative) language, which means what it says and says what it means; and (2) literary language, which we expect to be ambiguous. It includes metaphor, irony and the expectation that meaning will be elusive.[1] Practical language, the language of applied science, is useful for describing things and fixed concepts. Literary language is useful for both describing and even creating experience.

In strong contrast to so many other systems, devoted to ends external to themselves and their own processes, our style of therapy is a bit like literature, a continual exploration and reflection upon experience in all its forms; playing with the language of experience; a commentary on the validity of various ways of interpreting experience, an exploration of the creative, revelatory and deceptive powers of language (Culler, 2001, p. 35). In my therapeutic work I am always commenting on ways for integrating subjective experience, exploring how to make use of language so as to destabilize meaning in the interest of evoking possibility. This is a partial description of what I mean by "poetic knowing."

Until Carl Whitaker died in 1995, I had the pleasure of collaborating with him (e.g., see Whitaker & Keith, 1981; Keith & Whitaker, 1980, 1981, 1983a, 1983b; Denofsky, 2004).[2] After his death I started a project dedicated to him intending to write about clinical work with schizophrenia and families. The project bogged down for a number of reasons, and I began to focus more on the therapeutic process in his work. I asked myself what was it that Whitaker did with schizophrenics that made a difference? I figured out that what was critical was how he used language. I went on from there. In recent years I have come to believe that awareness of how to use language is more important than psychodynamics in experiential psychotherapy. *Experiential psychotherapy is a therapy beyond interpretation.* The paradigm for experiential psychotherapy is parallel play (Keith, 2015). Consider Derrida (1981, p. 14): "To risk meaning nothing is the beginning of play." In both the examples that follow, you will see me risking meaning nothing.

Clinical Illustration #1

The following clinical story is an example of attending to symbolic relationships rather than causal relationships in action. The therapeutic action is dependent on my appreciation of the loose hold that language has on the reality to which it attends, and gives evidence that the playful use of words can generate results not always predictable by the users. In play, words and the syntax in which they arrive can become destabilizing ambiguous events.

In my 45 years as a therapeutic psychiatrist I have done a lot of work as clinical consultant to primary-care physicians. One morning I was in the Family Medicine Department to work with the residents. Dr. Sayles, chair of the Family Medicine Department, was a good friend, and frequent co-therapist. He asked to talk to me about a family with whom he was working and described the following family situation. There were three middle-aged brothers managing a successful property management and real estate firm, but under the direction of their widowed 83-year-old mother. Their father, who had developed and directed this firm, had died three years previously. Their mother became the matriarchal CEO of the family business. She was vigorous but troubled. She had limited business experience, and in effect was dependent on them to give her direction in how to direct them. She was persistently distressed and called her sons repeatedly; about the business, about dealing with her dead husband's possessions. She was having trouble making decisions but resisted turning power over to her sons because her husband wanted her to take charge of the business after his death. She asked their advice but dismissed their suggestions. The sons asked Dr. Sayles to work with their mother to relieve her anxiety. Her status and the family's prominence made my friend uneasy. He wanted to include a psychiatrist, my very self, in the treatment. "No," said the sons, "she does not want psychiatric help. She does not 'believe' in psychiatrists." My doctor friend went ahead. He saw her twice, then told me about it that morning when I was there to do some consultative work with the residents.

He was unusually distressed when he reviewed her problems with me; a series of fairly concrete complaints about her sons' behavior, issues related to running the family business, and her attempt to maintain the business in the way her husband would have wanted.

I listened, then gave him a more elaborate version of the following: "You could say, 'This certainly is a difficult set of problems for you to be dealing with all by yourself. It sounds like you are stuck with being father, mother and CEO. And you are so isolated! I guess one solution would be to get a partner, a new husband maybe? One possibility is that I could marry you. But my wife wouldn't like that. I would have to divorce her first. I am not sure she would think much of the idea. Or, I could arrange for you to adopt me and make me the oldest son, but I know your sons would be upset if I tried to be their boss.'"

My physician friend chuckled, "Sure, Keith, you could say something like that, but not me."

Three weeks later: "Dave, do you remember me telling you about the family matriarch and you suggested I say something I didn't think I should say? Well I saw her ten days ago and near the end of the interview, I did not feel I was being helpful and I was upset with myself. I couldn't think, I felt frustrated again. Then I heard myself saying almost exactly what you suggested. [This is one of those *"You Said What?"* moments.] It just came out as we were approaching the end of another frustrating, for me, session. I could scarcely believe I was saying it. She just looked at me for a long silent moment, then changed the subject, as though I hadn't said anything. She decided not to make another appointment. I thought I had made a mistake and felt badly about what I said and angry with you for suggesting it. I thought about calling you up to give you hell for ruining my reputation. But three days ago, a week after the interview, her son called and said, 'I don't know how you did it, Doc, but our Mother is a different woman. The number of phone calls has dropped. She is so much easier to talk with, she just isn't as anxious as she was. Thanks so much.'"

Then, three months later, Dr. Sayles phoned to tell me that the matriarch made a $45,000 donation to the Department of Family Medicine so that a fund could be established as a way to teach young family physicians to do "What Dr. Sayles does." Obviously attending to symbolic rather than causal relations can do wonders for the "bottom line"!

Comment: This was an unexpectedly good outcome. But we could not be certain what he had done. When she was troubled, what did her behavior signify? How did I know to say what I did? I was being playful with language embedded in the syntax of symptoms and relationships. I am not sure where those comments came from except my long-term implicit awareness of symbolic and experiential family relational systems. Part of it came from my sense that she was alone. Part of it came from what I know of psychodynamics, especially family relational dynamics, part of it came from my parallel-play mindset, and part of it came from the almost physiological spontaneous logic of language. I will say more in a bit. My initial comment was based on my perception of a symbolic system, the family's Totality of Concerns, which cannot be articulated. My view is that my clumsy absurd remark affected her symbolic (subjective) organization; it had an extra-intellectual effect in the realm of symbolic experience and provided what turned out to be a refreshing immersion in absurdity. Perhaps he had inadvertently teased her in a way that refreshed her, in a way that no one had in a long time (Keith, 2015).

Teased her? Yes, I call it "Therapeutic Teasing." "Therapeutic Teasing?" What will the Omnipresent Clinical Overseers say? Like most of what is important in psychotherapy, therapeutic teasing is an art. "Art always penetrates the particular fissures in one's psychic life" (Greenblatt, 2011, p. 3). If not grounded in caring, this teasing can be harmful. But teasing with caring contains implicit respect for the other. It helps to escape the unproductive limits of reason and conventional logic. It disrupts the language in which an experiential conundrum is embedded and fixed. It temporarily sets conventional patterns aside. Teasing is a form of play. It risks meaning nothing.

What are the meta-messages that can go with teasing grounded in caring? It says to the patient, "You know how to think." It invites the patient into absurdity. Most know of it, but don't expect to encounter absurdity in a clinical context. I find that being playful in clinical situations is a way to acknowledge respect for the other.

Part of what makes these spontaneous remarks effective is that they speak to a symbolic reality. "What is that like?" you may ask. I will attempt to give some sense with the following eloquent and brief paragraph:

> Symbols are densely inscrutable.
>   A symbol is only a true symbol when it is inexhaustible and unlimited in its meaning, when it utters in its arcane (hieratic and magical) languages of hint and intimation something that cannot be set forth, that does not correspond to words. It has many faces and many thoughts

and in its remotest depths remains inscrutable…It is formed by organic process…and thus constitutionally different from complex and reducible allegories, parables, and similes…Symbols cannot be stated or explained, and, confronted by their secret meaning in its totality are powerless.

(Tarkovsky, 1986/2010, p. 47)

If you can appreciate and enjoy Tarkovsky's paragraph, you are moving toward the realm of poetic knowing.

This is to suggest that symbolic reality is fundamental to human experiencing. While it is both omnipresent and powerful, it is not readily accessible. This is so true of most reports of emotional experience. Symbolic reality is not easily embodied in practical language. Thus spontaneous remarks in literary language come closer to symbolic realities.

Spontaneous remarks are likely to happen when I feel stuck or blocked. They also happen when I am being inducted into a role I experience as inappropriate to the interactional context.

Clinical Illustration #2

The next illustration occurred in a Community Mental Health Center. Helen Davis, 50 and divorced, was referred to the County Mental Health Clinic by a primary-care physician who heard a case conference I did on the use of the family to deal with ambiguous health problems. The referral read, "multiple somatic complaints, prescription drug abuse … evaluate and treat." On the phone, he said he was not certain I could be of help. She had an 18-year history of decline from an upper middle-class living style. She had multiple hospitalizations for intractable depression, including electro-convulsive therapy, leading to extrusion from her family. When insurance ran out, she entered the state hospital system, where treatment of her chronic physical symptoms resulted in prescription drug addiction. Most recently she was discharged from a 30-day drug treatment program because of insufficient motivation for change. This followed a four-month hospitalization at a state hospital for depression. She was wearing out her welcome at the partial care center.

It was *not* a pleasure to meet Mrs. Davis. She came into the office whining and complaining. Her skin was dingy, appeared unwashed, her chopped-off hair was stringy and dirty. Her glasses were tilted at 30 degrees across her nose. Her worn black coat, pinned shut because of missing buttons, had a crusty cream-colored exclamation point down the right side that looked as though it had been made with an ice cream cone. The weather was cold and wet, but she was wearing only worn canvas shoes torn out over her bunions.

She entered my office and fell into a chair massaging her forehead with one hand. "Oh, doctor, you've got to help me. You've got to give me something. Five days I have had a headache and no relief. Dr. Rausch gave me an injection and it helped a little. Ohhhh, you've got to do something! Please give me a shot!"

I was angry with her immediately. She was not asking, she was demanding. My physician demeanor took over. No matter what the crisis, stay calm, be calming. I began in my usual way by taking a history. After only five sentences, she said, "Oh, I can't go on. I can't think. Ask my doctor to tell you all this. You've got to give me *something*!" She sobbed and held her hands to her head.

"I am sorry you are uncomfortable, Mrs. Davis, but I have to get this information in order to treat you appropriately."

Then she reset her posture to put some pressure on this uncooperative doctor. Here comes another "You Said What?" moment, this time interjected by the patient.

"Are you really a doctor? I mean what kind of a doctor? If you are really a doctor wouldn't you have a nicer office than this?" (I was working in the generic mental-health center physician's office. No diploma on the wall. Beat up over-used office furniture.) I stuck with my agenda and learned many had failed with her in the past.

She persisted. "Doctor, I need something. Aren't you going to give me something? I need some Valium or some Placidyl. You could give me a little Darvon, what's wrong with a little Darvon? I've been eating too much. You could give me some Dexamyl. You have to help me." I had the feeling she was like an old prizefighter, bobbing and weaving, jabbing desperately. I felt stuck. This bedraggled woman with tension headaches was a caricature of a patient. I was caught in a familiar but ridiculous situation in which the patient is saying, "Doctor, you're so powerful, help me, but you are too inadequate to do anything."

Frustration is a stimulus for creativity. I had an idea.

"I realize I am being difficult. I do want to help you. But I don't want to repeat the errors of others."

"Well then, what are you going to do?"

Here comes the "*You Said What?*" moment. "This is going to be difficult. *I am going to teach you how to suffer.*"

She exploded. "What! Teach me how to suffer? But I am already suffering."

"I know, but you are no good at it. You have been suffering many years, but you keep thinking there is a solution. Learning how to suffer means that you give up believing there is an end to it. You stop going back to the solutions that don't work."

Now she was furious. "I can't believe this. This is just stupid. You're going to teach me how to *suffer*?"

I became a caricature of a caring physician responding to her caricature of a patient. She became angry with me and incredulous. I urged her not to be angry with me, but to try and see how much I wanted to help her. But further, I warned her I would be totally useless unless she brought her daughter to the next visit in five days. My standard move when confronted with difficult clinical situations is to add people on either side of the therapeutic relationship. Mrs. Davis was in this city because her daughter was attending the university here.

She came to the next appointment with her daughter. Vicki was a pleasant 22-year-old woman who contrasted sharply with her mother. She was clear-skinned, bright-eyed and unpretentious. Her manner reflected both concern for her mother as well as peevishness.

Her daughter was supportive of my efforts. However, I had destabilized the situation and an undercurrent of urgency emerged. I knew that any new pressure would be imposed on Vicki's shoulders. In order to help Vicki deal with the instability introduced by me, I suggested they return in three days. Vicki agreed over her mother's objection. I was assuming the daughter could be a partial solution for her mother's profound problems. But I know that in work with chronic illness any solution can be transformed into being part of the problem.

When they returned, Mrs. Davis was furious. She complained loudly during the hour that I was not being helpful to her. She cried because she felt hopeless that there was anyone who could help her. However, she looked brighter. Her hair was clean, her coat was open and the white exclamation point was gone. She said the sessions were doing no good. "I am suffering more than I was before I came." I told her I was glad to hear my treatment was going so well so soon. "It sounds like you have already given up hope, and I think that's a marvelous step forward for you." She said she hated me and that her headaches became much worse during the hours before she came to the clinic. She did not want to come back. Her daughter said, "Mother, he is doing what you need. I wish we had met him long ago."

They returned, and I worked with them for two and a half years. It is an interesting story. There were a number of important therapeutic events. Initially Helen became more sociable; for a time she had a romantic relationship with a male patient, about ten years her junior. Vicki didn't approve. Helen was like a 13-year-old daughter in love in the middle of puberty, and Vicki became mother-like. Helen soon became disenchanted with the 'boy' friend. "I don't know what I was thinking," she confessed. Someone gave Helen an old sewing machine; she got some clothing from the Salvation Army store and refashioned it to fit her and to make it more fashionable. She surprised me with her talent. The whole story is summarized in an article that appeared in *Family Process* in 1980, "The Case of Helen D.: A Woman Who Learned to Suffer" (Keith, 1980).

I am writing about it here because my *"You Said What?"* remark was completely spontaneous, in the moment. I had never done that before, nor have I used that same line since. Much of what we regard as "mental illness" is role-determined. She was in the role of demanding, chronically mentally-ill patient seeking someone to be in the supporting cast. I surprised myself by what I said, but her response helped me to stay in a therapeutic groove; her role complemented mine. I have not read anything about psychodrama, but this might be considered spontaneous psychodrama. It is a bit like "improv" where the actor has responsibility for the other actors who are also the audience.

Others find it hard to do this. They are amused or impressed by what I am doing, they try it and it does not work, or it has a negative effect. I suspect that is true because they are too intentional, too purposeful. It also will have no effect if the therapist is anxious. When an anxious mother seeks to soothe a baby, the baby cries harder, activated by her anxiety. They may not know enough about their own sadism, and there is too much sadism in their actions.

I mentioned assuming my physician role setting a structure for our interaction. It is very important. The more upset they get, the calmer I become. That is a role I learned to play and I play it well. We arranged with a local community theater to give our residents acting lessons. I expected we would be taught how to develop a character based on who that person was. But no. They gave us dialogue to do. In character we were to decide what we wanted from the other. That is what guided how we delivered our lines. What did we want from the other?

There are three fundamental and implicit components to an experiential therapy interaction: empathy, caring, and attention.

Attention: There is a kind of attention that has emotional energy in it. Children are nurtured by this kind of attention. An anxious parent provides attention, but the attention agitates the child (Keith, 2015).

Empathy: Empathy can be characterized as the ability to imaginatively enter into the experience of others. Believe it or not, these "You Said What?" moments are grounded in empathy. Empathy is fundamental to our nature as social beings. I think of empathy as occurring in a system modeled after the peripheral nervous system. There are afferent (incoming) tracts and efferent (outgoing) tracts. In the therapeutic context, empathy is a process where we receive (via afferent tracts) large quantities of not-categorical information, largely nonverbal, from an Other. The information reverberates in us and we feed it back (via efferent tracts) with sensitivity that is nuanced for the situation. Empathy is a subjective experience, stimulated by the presence of an Other, or group of related Others (a family), and the interaction that emerges is unique to therapy with this family at this particular time.

Empathy might take the form of giving a name to the apparent feelings of another ("You look discouraged"). It might mean responding to someone who appears sad by putting a hand on their shoulder. I refer to this conventional characterization of empathy as *Supportive Empathy*.

In experiential therapy, oriented around growth and change, we want empathy to be *therapeutic*. Thus, we take the input and go one step further by letting the emotional experience reverberate in us and then give back our response, even when apparently non-congruent or ironic, in an effort to induce something like destabilization, in order to nudge them out of their normal. Empathy of this sort will (hopefully) induce transient disruption of a stuck situation. This second type of empathy is *Therapeutic Empathy*. It pressures for destabilization in the interest of increasing the possibility for change and expansion of health (Keith, 2015).

Caring: I have mentioned caring throughout the essay. I will be brief: *in the therapeutic relationship caring is a form of love without hunger.*

Attention + Empathy = Caring

In this therapy pattern we are hoping to alter the patient/family consciousness of their world by distorting/contaminating their orientation, another name for destabilization. Supportive empathy, which reflects or placates, or is stimulated by a therapist's need to be helpful, can inadvertently entrench the patient if the feeling state is reified, made into a something. I have tried to give some sense of where those *"You Said What?"* moments come from. But my essay is an abbreviated, only suggestive summary. There is much more to say. I hope I have aroused your curiosity so that you learn to think more deeply about your work as therapist.

Reflection

I will end with a short story from the early 70s when I first met Carl Whitaker. Carl had done a weekend workshop with Salvador Minuchin. Both were pioneering founders and innovators in the family therapy world. Minuchin (1974) developed Structural Family Therapy, which was eminently teachable. It became and still is very popular; probably the most coherent, influential, and user-friendly family therapy method. They shared a warm mutual appreciation.[2] After the workshop Minuchin told Whitaker he was fascinated with what Carl did in the therapy interview. But the problem with it, he said, is that Whitaker's methods "can't be taught." Carl was slightly dispirited by this assessment. Then a month or so later Carl articulated a new aphorism which became a mantra, *"What's worth knowing can't be taught. It must be learned"* (Keith, 2015).

Notes

1 "[U]nderstanding consists in reducing one type of reality to another; that the true reality is never the most obvious; and that the nature of truth is already indicated by the care it takes to remain elusive" (Jonathan Culler, 2001, p. 27).

2 For some of Whitaker's other writing, see Whitaker (1958, 1982, 1989); Whitaker and Bumberry (1988); Whitaker and Malone (1953); Whitaker and Napier (1978).

3 A few years later, in his Foreword to Whitaker's collected papers, Minuchin (1982, p. ix) wrote: "Any statement presented as complete is turned into a fragment. Like James Joyce, Whitaker creates a revolution in the grammar of life ... Whitaker's assumption seems to be that out of his challenge to form, creative processes in individual family members as well as the family as a whole can arise ... By the end of therapy, every family member has been touched by Whitaker's distorting magic. Each member feels challenged, misunderstood, accepted, rejected, or insulted. But he has been put in contact with a less familiar part of himself."

References

Culler, J. (2001). *The pursuit of signs: Semiotics, literature, deconstruction.* Ithaca, NY: Cornell University Press.

Denofsky, H. (2004). *Clinical dialogues in family therapy, based on the psychotherapy of Carl Whitaker, M. D. and David Keith, M. D.* Frederick, MD: PubishAmerica.

Derrida, J. (1981). *Positions.* (A. Bass, Trans). Chicago, IL: University of Chicago Press.

Greenblatt, S. (2011). *The swerve: How the world became modern.* New York: Norton.

hooks, b. (1995). *Art on my mind: Visual politics.* New York: New Press.

Keith, D. V. (1980). The case of Helen D.: A woman who learned to suffer. *Family Process, 19,* 269–275.

Keith, D. V. (2015). *Continuing the experiential approach of Carl Whitaker: Process, practice & magic.* Phoenix, AZ: Zeig, Tucker & Theisen.

Keith, D. V., & Kaye, D. L. (2001). Consultation with the extended family: Primary process in clinical practice. *Child and Adolescent Psychiatric Clinics of North America, 10*(3), 563–576.

Keith, D. V., & Whitaker, C. A. (1980). Add craziness and stir: Psychotherapy with a psychoticogenic family. In: M. Andolfi & I. Zwerling (Eds.). *Dimensions in family therapy* (pp. 139–160). New York: Guilford Press.

Keith, D. V., & Whitaker, C. A. (1981). Play therapy: A paradigm for work with families. *Journal of Marital and Family Therapy. 7,* 243–254.

Keith, D. V., & Whitaker, C. A. (1983a). Cotherapy with families. In B. Wolman & G. Stricker (Eds.). *Handbook of family and marital therapy* (pp. 343–355). New York: Plenum Press.

Keith, D. V., & Whitaker, C. A. (1983b). Failure: Our bold companion. In S. Coleman (Ed.). *Failure in family therapy* (pp. 8–23). New York: Guilford Press.

Minuchin, S. (1974). *Families and family therapy.* Cambridge, MA: Harvard University Press.

Minuchin, S. (1982). Foreword. In J. R. Neill & D. P. Kniskern (Eds.). *From psyche to system: The evolving therapy of Carl Whitaker* (pp. vii–ix). New York: Guilford Press.

Prosky, P. S., & Keith, D. V. (Eds.). (2003). *Family therapy as an alternative to medication: An appraisal of Pharmland.* New York: Routledge.

Tarkovsky, A. (2010). *Sculpting in time: Reflections on the cinema.* Austin, TX: University of Texas Press. (Originally published in 1986.)

Whitaker, C. A. (1958). *Psychotherapy with chronic schizophrenic patients.* Boston: Little, Brown.

Whitaker, C. A. (1976). The hindrance of theory in clinical work. In P. J. Guerin (Ed.). *Family therapy: Theory and practice.* New York: Gardner Press. Reprinted in *From Psyche to System: The evolving therapy of Carl Whitaker* (pp. 317–329; J. R. Neill & D. P. Kniskern, Eds.). New York: Guilford Press.

Whitaker, C. A. (1982). *From psyche to system: The evolving therapy of Carl Whitaker* (pp. 317–329; J. R. Neill & D. P. Kniskern, Eds.). New York: Guilford Press.

Whitaker, C. A. (1989). *Midnight musings of a family therapist.* (M. O. Ryan, Ed.). New York: Norton.

Whitaker, C. A., & Bumberry, W. M. (1988). *Dancing with the family: A symbolic-experiential approach.* Bristol, PA: Brunner/Mazel.

Whitaker, C. A., & Keith, D. (1981). Symbolic-experiential family therapy. In A. Gurman & D. Kniskern (Eds.). *The handbook of family therapy*. New York: Brunner/ Mazel. Reprinted in *From psyche to system: The evolving therapy of Carl Whitaker* (pp. 330–363; J. R. Neill & D. P. Kniskern, Eds.). New York: Guilford Press.

Whitaker, C. A., & Malone, T. (1953). *The roots of psychotherapy*. New York: Blakiston.

Whitaker, C., A., & Napier, A. Y. (1978). *The family crucible*. New York: Harper & Row.

CHAPTER 15

When Impatience Gets the Best of Me

Jeffrey Kottler

Let's acknowledge that I'm not the most patient person. I became a therapist in the first place under the misguided notion that I could fix other people's problems because I felt so helpless to deal with some of my own issues. I suppose impatience is one of those at the top of the list.

Under the best of circumstances, I'm in a hurry to get things done. My inbox is usually empty. I respond to correspondence or messages within hours, if not minutes (I wrote this chapter within hours of receiving the invitation). Sometimes I think that those "close door" buttons on elevators or buttons on crosswalks were invented just for me – even though they rarely seem to work (I've wondered if they aren't really just decoys to give us something to do while waiting).

I've always felt life is short and anything worth doing can be done quickly and more efficiently. I suppose many others must agree with me, considering that we now have speed dating, 7-minute workouts apps, and even speed yoga.

I'm a fast walker, usually in front of the pack during climbs, hikes, or treks. It's therefore not surprising that, although I was originally trained in psychodynamic and existential therapy, I immediately jumped on the brief therapy bandwagon – that is until I realized how many more referrals I would need to remain in practice.

Over time I've learned to moderate myself, to proceed at the often glacial pace of some of my clients who want to take their time thinking about all kinds of things before they ever move into action mode. "That's okay," I repeatedly reassure myself, "they will move forward when they're ready."

A Lost Cause

Not unlike contemporary times when the opioid addictions have become a major public health threat, the 1980s were dominated by cocaine as the intoxicant of choice, at least among the affluent who could afford such an indulgence. Psychotherapy isn't exactly very effective – or long-lasting – in treating any addiction, but with respect to treating cocaine users it was next to worthless. The high was just too enticing, the drug too powerful to quit.

I'd had poor luck (or skills) attempting to treat other drug addictions with weekly therapy as the singular option, but with respect to cocaine users, sessions were absolutely worthless. Clients would make all kinds of promises and the commitment wouldn't last beyond a day or two. I had exhausted every strategy, technique, intervention, or method within my repertoire in such cases and failed miserably every time.

I agreed to see a new referral when he told me on the phone he was having some family issues. That sounded both familiar and relatively benign, the sort of thing I could "fix" within a relatively short period of time. I already had a full caseload, mostly of relatively long-term clients, so I was eager to work with someone who might show immediate improvement.

Nigel seemed like the embodiment of a successful business executive. Expensive suit. Tie loosened at the collar. Rolex watch. Haughty attitude.

As soon as he walked in I found that I didn't like him very much.

"How can I help you?" I began right away. He seemed like the type of guy who would say something like, "Time is money."

"Well, as I mentioned on the phone, I'm sort of having some family problems."

"Family problems?" I prompted, settling into the familiar routine.

"Yeah," he shrugged. "Mostly my wife."

"So, you're having some marital issues," I clarified.

Another shrug.

I waited. Maybe it was punitive on my part. As I said, I resented the man's seeming arrogance and obvious affluence.

Nigel sighed, as if to communicate this was a bit more complicated than he first indicated.

"Actually, maybe my wife is the one who should be seeing you. She's the one who is upset about things."

"What things?" Now I was intrigued. There was something going on here that wasn't quite as it seemed. My impatience was rearing its head.

"I suppose you've heard this sort of thing before. My wife thinks I have some sort of drug problem or something."

"Or something?"

"Okay. She is worried about me."

I waited. And waited. Finally, I added: "Because ..."

"I do a little cocaine from time to time. Nothing too excessive. Just a few lines when I need it. I have a very stressful job. Lots of responsibility. People depend on me."

"I see," I said. And I did see. I had been seeing this sort of thing a lot lately.

"It's really no big deal," he was quick to point out.

"So, let me see if I understand what you are saying. Your wife thinks you have a serious drug problem that is both dangerous and affecting your relationship, not to mention other aspects of your life. But, you think she is just overreacting, that you have everything under control. And the cocaine is not really a problem. Does that about cover it?"

Nigel could tell I wasn't exactly buying his version of the story. It turned out, after pressing for details, he admitted that he was going through a gram of cocaine each day, hitting lines every few hours to fuel his energy and confidence in the face of unremitting pressures. For the first time, I felt some compassion for the guy, realizing just what his world must be like, the appearances that must be kept up, the difficulties he was facing. I was also struck by his denial and image management. I kept looking at him and wondering what I could possibly say or do that would make any difference. Whereas Nigel seemed to be putting on a good show of confidence and optimism, actually believing I had some answer for him, all I could feel was despair and helplessness.

In my mind, I reviewed the catalogue of anything I might try, any strategy that I might introduce with this case and came up empty. Sure, I'd had some success at times with people addicted to bad habits, even substances, but so far, I'd never put a dent in anyone who was using cocaine on a daily basis, especially someone wealthy enough to afford it. I considered – and rejected – anything I could offer to this man that might be helpful. We could examine the conditions and circumstances of his life that led to his need for a chemical crutch to manage his anxiety. We could spend time talking about his history and background. I could try to get him to join a 12-step program. I could even refer him to an inpatient facility to detoxify. But none of those options had ever worked before, at least for very long. And especially with someone who wouldn't admit he had a problem in the first place. His incentive to alter his behavior was minimal, except for empty threats by his wife. His motivation to change his patterns, or even reduce his dependency on the drug, was minimal: he kept insisting he didn't really have a problem.

When I asked Nigel what I could do for him, or what he wanted from me, he just kind of shrugged. He had made it clear the only reason he showed up in the first place was because his wife insisted he see someone to talk about this.

I looked at my watch and noticed that only 20 minutes of the session had elapsed. Yet I knew, I just *knew*, that talking to him further was a colossal waste of time for both of us. I was not only feeling impatient but also bored by this interaction, because I could see where it was going and where we would end up. And it wasn't pretty. I'd been through this with so many others in previous months and the outcome was always hopeless.

Nigel was still waiting for me to offer some reassurance that he was indeed correct, his wife wrong, and he didn't really have a problem. He was used to being in control, directing how such conversations went, and he seemed to be proud of the way he had managed me.

Maybe I was just tired, or in a bad mood. Certainly, I was feeling impatient. (These are the best excuses I can muster after the fact.) I just looked at Nigel and shook my head.

"What?" he asked, perhaps more stridently than he intended.

I hesitated, wondering if I should really say what I was thinking out loud.

"What?" he insisted.

Deep breath. "Nigel. Nigel. Nigel. I can't help you."

"You can't?"

"Nope. Nobody can. You have a serious physiological addiction, and psychological dependence, on one of the most dangerous drugs you can find."

"But I know lots of people who ..."

I held up my hand to stop him. "Please let me finish. You asked me what I think, so now I'm going to tell you. And you aren't going to like it. You're not even going to listen to me, much less believe what I'm about to tell you. But, here goes anyway.

"As I was saying, the nature of your addiction to this drug, the amount you are consuming on a daily basis, qualifies as rather extreme. You are spending thousands of dollars each month just to maintain your habit. You are probably noticing it takes more and more to get the same high. You are hiding your behavior from everyone, lying to your family, friends, and colleagues, and mostly to yourself. I just can't help you. Your prognosis is terrible."

"So, what are you saying?" his voice rising in indignation. "You won't help me?"

"No, what I'm saying is that I *can't* help you." I looked at my watch again, as if to say that we were done even though the session was just half over.

Nigel looked down and shook his head. I wasn't sure if this gesture signaled disappointment in me or disgust in himself. He looked up momentarily and held up his palm, asking me to continue with anything else. "So, that's it? Nothing to be done? Nothing else you can offer me? No hope?"

Now, here it comes. This is the "*Said WHAT?*" moment. This is the challenging situation in which I tried something for the first time, not so much creative as desperate, reflecting my frustration and impatience.

"Look, Mr. G. (I had now reverted to formalities as I was dismissing him). "You want to know what the cure is for your condition? You want to know what will fix this? Okay, here it is. You will escalate to doing even more cocaine. Then you'll start to act out in even more extreme ways – sexually, risk-taking, decision-making, impulsive behavior. The cost of your habit will skyrocket out of control until you can no longer afford to hide the extent of what you're doing. You will be so far in debt you'll probably end up in bankruptcy. You'll lose your job. Your marriage will end. Your kids will blame you for everything and it will take you the rest of your life to repair the damage. When, or *if*, you ever recover after you've lost everything, you'll still have some chronic health problems that will take years off your lifespan – that is, if you don't die of abuse or an overdose sooner rather than later."

After I said my spiel, Nigel was understandably stunned. This was not at all what he expected from our encounter. "So, that's it?" he finally asked after a long silence.

"Sorry, but yes, that's it. I can't help you."

Nigel stood up with dignity, shook my hand, and thanked me for my trouble. Then he calmly walked out the door. I still had 15 minutes left in the session to consider how inappropriate, unprofessional, and wildly shocking my behavior had been. I wondered if it might be time to take a break from this work?

A Parallel Process

This interaction was actually part of a pattern that emerged during this time in my life and career when I was feeling burned out by private practice. I had lost some of my passion. I was tired of working with the relatively affluent worried well. I was tired of listening to the complaints of people who were mostly bored with the routines and emptiness of their lives. Of course, there was a parallel process going on in which that's exactly what *I* was feeling in my own predicament. This led to considerable soul-searching and a decision to quit what I was doing and rededicate myself to public service and working with indigent clients. In some small way, Nigel helped push me in this direction. I felt like I wasn't being very useful.

I don't hold out this case as a stellar example of "creative therapy in challenging situations." On the contrary, I've co-edited a number of volumes (e.g., Kottler, 2017; Kottler & Carlson, 2003, 2008, 2009, 2015) of such seminal stories from the most famous living theoreticians and practitioners, and almost every one of the narratives appeared to describe some brilliant breakthrough that resulted from the therapists' superior wisdom, experience, and inventiveness. Not a single one resulted from laziness, frustration, or impatience.

Comment

The clinical choices I made were not necessarily in the best interests of my client. I reacted somewhat impulsively and impatiently. I consider my actions to have been both risky and perilous, mostly as a result of my own frustration and personal issues going on at the time. So many of my clients were making small, incremental changes in their lives that took months for visible results in evidence. I was hungry, even desperate, to feel more potent, more useful, and I jumped on these cases as opportunities to say some of the things I'd been holding back for a long time. I don't hold up this case as exemplary of creative work. Instead, it is a reminder for me to pay closer attention to my own personal needs, as well as how they may play out in my relationships with clients.

Follow Up

I hesitate to mention the end of this story for fear that it will dilute the message. But here goes. Perhaps I wouldn't have had the courage to share it if the outcome were unknown or uncertain. I have thought about it for over 30 years. I always wondered what happened to that guy. And on some level, I have held on to regret about the way I behaved with him. Even more disturbing, I worried that I had done him serious harm when he was so desperate to reach out for a lifeline. Instead I had left him to drown. I learned a lot from that interaction. I have made a point to allow myself to feel remorse. I use that experience as a reminder to monitor carefully my impatience and frustration, and to access greater compassion, even when my own sense of helplessness is triggered.

A few years ago, one of my brothers told me a story that has given me pause and polishes the end of the story. My brother still lives in the city where I grew up and once practiced earlier in my career. It's not unusual that he runs into one of my ex-clients who recognizes his last name and asks him to pass on their regards.

"So," my brother reported to me, "I ran into this guy, one of your ex-clients. His name is Nigel G-."

Silence from me. He knows I won't acknowledge whether someone was ever my client and he thinks that's amusing.

"He wanted me to say 'Hi.' He had this amazing story to tell about you."

"Oh yeah?" I answered, partly apprehensive, partly curious.

"Apparently he came to see you one time. You didn't even let him finish the session. You told him he was a hopeless case."

"Oh shit," I thought. "NOW I'm in trouble. He tracked me down through my brother and now there will be hell to pay. Heck, I probably deserve it."

I held my breath waiting for the rest.

"Anyway, you scared him to death. You told him he was going to lose everything in his life and there was nothing he could do until he lost it all." My brother was laughing as he said this. "Did you *really* tell him that?"

I didn't answer.

"So, Nigel tells me when he left your office he got inside his car and started crying. He was absolutely terrified. He had a vial of coke in his glove compartment and he reached inside for it."

Holy crap! Now I was really worried. I drove the guy into greater despair!

"But, then you scared the shit out of him so badly that he opened the window and threw the vial away. He told me from that moment he never touched the stuff again. Went cold turkey. Anyway, he wanted me to thank you for what you did."

You just never know.

References

Kottler, J. (2017). *Secrets of exceptional counselors*. Alexandria, VA: American Counseling Association.

Kottler, J., & Carlson, J. (2003). *The mummy at the dining room table: Eminent therapists reveal their most unusual cases and what they teach us about human behavior*. San Francisco: Jossey-Bass.

Kottler, J., & Carlson, J. (2008). *Their finest hour: Master therapists share their greatest success stories*. Bethel, CT: Crown House Publishers.

Kottler, J., & Carlson, J. (2009). *Creative breakthroughs in therapy: Tales of transformation and astonishment*. New York: Wiley.

Kottler, J., & Carlson J. (2015). *On being a master therapist: Practicing what we preach*. New York: Wiley.

CHAPTER 16

The Single Stroke
What Makes "Zingers" Zing?[1]
Michele Ritterman

A single stroke of the brush does not work a miracle for every client. Each person, couple, family, community is unique. As such, every case we treat requires a one-of-a-kind method of problem solving. Picasso, for example, with very few lines limned the shape of a young woman and it is perfect as it is. One or two strokes, and a world evoked – Woman! Youth! Sensuality! But he also painted *Guernica*, to tell a different story, that of the horrors of fascism, and for that, he needed many lines and forms and colors.

As healers, we will be called upon to do what is necessary at any one moment with any given client. Most important is to understand the client response, more than the therapist intervention. Then we can grasp how the clear representation of the needed image or words, at exactly the right moment and interjected with laser-beam accuracy into the correct spot, sometimes can be as David's stone was destructive for Goliath and as healing as Cupid's arrow to the heart.

In my experience, to make therapy a single stroke – the simplest, most straightforward statement, suggestion, or question – actually requires a complex understanding of a person's presenting trouble or symptom. The better our understanding, the more likely we are to be granted the client's attention and to foster receptivity to the message we hope will be useful.

A Tri-Level Model to Identify a Quick Intervention

To find that exact moment and precisely receptive spot, one way is to look for the world in the therapy room. Each person/couple/family is a zoom lens into a slice of the life of the world today, of a specific community, of a set of values and agreements both outside and inside themselves. I often like to start wide-angle and zoom in from the world/society, to the intimate relationships that may pertain, and finally to the self- or body-talk that holds a symptom in a stuck place.

My first book, *Using Hypnosis in Family Therapy* (1983/2005), was a systematic integration of Erickson-style hypnotherapy and family therapy *à la* Jay

Haley and Salvador Minuchin, and Braulio Montalvo. I opened (2005, pp. 2–3) with this example of *Three Levels of Symptom Induction:*

A well-dressed Spanish-speaking woman is brought by her friend to an outpatient clinic. She has not been able to stop crying for four months. She is alone, she is pregnant, and she feels that she is incapable of having a child in her present state. However, since the thought of abortion makes her feel like a murderer, she believes she should die. This first level of her situation – the individual mind-set she is trapped in – causes irreconcilable conflict between what she feels like doing and what she believes she should do. According to her present way of thinking, she can kill the baby or kill herself – or cry continuously. Her symptom "all I can do is cry" seems her way of avoiding the other choices.

Consider the second level of her situation – her family context. How does her symptom reflect this aspect of her life? We learn that the woman had recently married a young doctor in Central America. They had decided to have a child together, but suddenly, without warning, he was missing, and she fled to the United States, leaving parents and friends behind. Clearly, her symptom of crying denotes her terrible loss of power, control, and meaning in terms of family life and family development. She had married a man of prominence but is now a widow, and pregnant ...

The woman's symptom also reflects a third level or aspect of her life – her social context. The woman had been a devout Catholic in El Salvador, where abortion is considered unthinkable, the greatest sin. Truly, in her social situation, she is bereft of all sense of personal power and meaning in life. Catholicism was her source of philosophy about the world, yet she is aching to not bring a child into the world. This third facet of her symptom intersects with her options of despair and loss of family supports, producing a convergence of negative positions in all her hierarchies of meaning and doing. All she can do is cry.

If the woman had a different mental attitude, family developmental situation, religious perspective or social context, she might not manifest symptoms, although she might be grievous. As things stand, her symptom is best regarded as the point where all three contexts that she temporarily inhabits converge in suggesting hopelessness.

How do we even get her attention, which is the first step to delivering a successfully received zing or mind-opener? I said to her: "There are not tears enough for your situation. Surely yours is the life God chose for you to go on to represent your heroic family and religion. Is it not true that 'To save one life is to save the world'? And that the whole Bible can be reduced to two words: *Choose Life.*"

I had used her own profound – if shaken – faith. I had acknowledged her pain and met her in her worldview. I got her attention. She awoke from her tears and looked directly at me.

I continued: "Will you help me help you keep your family alive first by helping you as a Catholic and humanist to save your own life?"

She nodded as she listened. We could then go back in time to talk about her pregnancy: "If so, let's start by bringing into our experience your family and community that were originally part of your decision to bring a baby into the world. When and where was the decision to have a child made?"

In this era of obsession with diagnoses and drugs which regards the individual seeking our help as the primary unit of focus, we must remember to bring their world into the therapy session and our interventions. The best thing a student ever said to me was: "Thank you. You taught me that the world is represented in the therapy room."

Healing Over Time: The Artistry of They Did What, You Said What, and How Did They Respond?

How does the therapist learn about the client, in order to say that one right thing? First, by tracking sequences of interaction (thought or thought and behavior) that are natural to that client – this can happen quickly or over time. And then, by inserting your single stroke and watching what happens.

I worked like this for many years before my teacher, Braulio Montalvo, sent me the videotape *Rivers and Tides: Andy Goldsworthy Working with Time* (Riedelman, 2001) and wrote: "Andy Goldsworthy, the artist, does his art just like you do your therapy." As I learned from the tape and subsequent reading and viewing (Goldsworthy, 2000; Riedelman, 2018), Goldsworthy is a Scottish-born artist who specializes in working with natural materials (e.g., stones, leaves, ice) to track and evoke the passage of time. Like Goldsworthy, I look at the natural resources that are already there in the person/couple/family, seeing how interactional sequences flow naturally – collecting the stones and flowers, the sunlight and the tides, seeing how the autumn leaves begin to drop from a tree – from one spontaneous event to another, then I insert my one-liner. The goal is to watch what the client does with the one-liner: THAT is what matters – just as Goldsworthy watches to see what nature will do with what he did with the natural environment. Therein lies the artful healing. There is no quick fix: Love and healing take time. Hate harms. Caring can repair (Ritterman, 2009, pp. 74–75). Express yourself clearly, then see what happens.

Two Cases in Which a Few Strokes of Intervention Affected Multiple Levels of a Person's Symptom in One Fell Swoop

A few lines made the difference. Would that I could more often find such a laser beam for everyone, especially myself. But not all situations so nicely connect the social unit, the family dynamic and the experience of a personal trouble.

Case Example. In one couple I saw, the husband was a Quaker and not allowed to manifest overt anger. He told his wife that he couldn't read her mind, but if she would directly ask him, he would be glad to help with household chores.

When his wife of many years asked him to do any of the tasks he'd overtly agreed to as part of running the household, he would say "Yes" or "Sure," but then not do the task. The wife claimed that after she made any request he also became angry with her as though he were being put upon, and that he would be passively punishing: not talking to her, not showing affection, acting as if she had said he was a bad boy when she felt she was just asking him to be the helpful husband.

A typical incident arose, and I observed him carefully, to see whether she was right or not, about what happened inside of him. After doing so, I asked:

"Your wife just asked you to take out the trash. How do you feel about that?"

"Fine," he said.

"No resentment or anger toward her?"

He said, "Definitely not – it's a perfect example of her reading into things."

"OK," I said. "Would you like to know more about yourself? Sometimes we hide things even from ourselves because we don't approve of our feelings."

"Sure," he said, "nothing to hide over here!"

"OK, are you absolutely certain you'd like to know more about yourself, even if it might make you feel a little uncomfortable?"

"Sure," he said again. "Absolutely."

"OK. Then, without disturbing your two hands at all – do not move them yet – I'd like you to super slowly remove your left hand from where it sits on top of your right hand. Leaving your right hand exactly as it is now."

He looked down at his hands as if he'd never seen them before. He slowly lifted his left from his right, and we all saw the white knuckled fist his right hand was still forming.

"What's that?" I asked, eager to see how my intervention would affect his use of his own natural resources.

"Wow," he said. "I had no idea ..."

"That's right," I said. "That's good to know, isn't it? And now you know what your wife is experiencing."

This was the start of a different discourse and ultimately a positive conclusion for the couple: That in their home, it was OK for him to learn to say "Yes" and "No," to experience himself as a peer of his wife, to step up to the plate (and sink!), but not feel dominated, and for the wife to trust her intuitions without feeling turned off to the husband.

The one-liner invitation, "Would you like to know more about yourself?," can help to *make the unconscious conscious.* Although many have emphasized Erickson's skills at helping people go into trance, I found Erickson was as much about helping a person do what I call "Breaking the Spell of a Dysfunctional Rapport" (Ritterman, 1985), that is, helping the person to wake up from a destructive trance. As described elsewhere (Ritterman, 2013, 2014, in press), Erickson was my main mentor. My studies with him began while I was still an intern at the Philadelphia Child Guidance Clinic and continued after I had moved to Seattle and then to Berkeley, finally interrupted by his death in 1980. Early in my training with Erickson, during a family session, I realized that the identified patient's symptoms were being induced by hypnotic suggestions embedded in the family interaction. The symptoms were the "automatic behavior" resulting from observable suggestions! I went to Erickson as soon as possible with my revelation: "Milton, family and society are the 24/7 ongoing daily hypnotists and symptoms are just trance states. We need to track the inductions for the symptoms trance and counter them with our systemic hypnosis." He gazed at me and said: *"If I were you, I'd develop that idea."* The well-placed single-stroke zinger is good for that: it creates a surprise or shock that effectively says, "WAKE UP!" I prefer that we help people TO AWAKEN, so that they feel not only relieved of their problems but also empowered to see themselves as the source of their improvement.

Another Case Example. I remember that once while I was with Erickson in his office during our precious time together, the desk phone rang. I couldn't hear the speaker on the other side, but only Erickson.

"Severely obese? And you've done what so far?" There was a long stretch it seemed when he listened and looked pensive.

"So you've seen tens of therapists over the years and they've all failed you? How far away is your grocery store? Have you ever bought your food for the week and walked back carrying it to see just the weight of it? Have you tried something in the store you never ate before? … Well, don't call me again until you do and don't waste my time." And he hung up.

I realized what his message was. Erickson had a file of letters from therapist bashers that he kept in the closet of the guest room where I slept when I visited. There are people who go to a therapist more to prove that therapists can't help them than to receive good advice. He sensed this person was like that. As Braulio Montalvo had said, the great clinician rejects the impossible cases at the phone call. Erickson was telling this woman that she needed to take charge of the situation herself if she was to receive help from him. And that first she had to break the stream of prior events in which empathic clinicians may have been suckered into unintentionally supporting her habit of overeating. His interest was to convey there wouldn't be a minute of that with him. Don't waste MY time. Really also meaning "Stop wasting YOUR time; and don't call me until you do." He left the door open.

Many years later I was doing work on behalf of Amnesty International and the American Family Therapy Association against state-sanctioned torture which was pervasive under the Pinochet dictatorship in Chile (see Ritterman, 1987). At that moment, I was trying to help one political prisoner attain liberation before he would be put under death sentence and be placed in a deprivation chamber until the execution. As described in my book *Hope Under Siege: Terror and Family Support in Chile* (Ritterman, 1991), there were 15 such people. I received many strange calls during that time. Don't get me wrong, I am a big believer in love and caring. At the risk of sounding overly sentimental,

I will say that great therapy is guided by feelings of love and, in what follows, like Erickson's, my one-liner might not sound loving but it was.

One time late in the afternoon I got a phone call in my office in Berkeley. The person said: "I have decided to kill myself, and I want you to help me commit suicide."

"If you are going to kill yourself, why would you call me for that?" I asked, a bit shocked and also sensing something disingenuous in his voice, as Erickson had detected in his caller.

"Life has no meaning for me."

I felt that same manipulation Erickson had heard.

"Great!" I said. "I already have a plan for you."

"What?" he said, clearly surprised that I had so quickly taken the bait.

"Yes. I can help you commit suicide!" I said with great faux-enthusiasm.

"You what?" The caller was now in shock.

"If you will fly with me to Santiago, Chile and immolate yourself outside of the Public Prison, like the monks did during the war in Vietnam, you could save the lives of 15 political prisoners!"

"Why ... but why ..." (Now I had the person's attention.) "But then ... would my life have meaning?"

"Yes. Great meaning."

"Then why would I want to commit suicide?"

"Exactly!" I said. "And thanks for calling. Please don't hesitate to call me back if you are interested."

"Thank you."

I had sensed that my natural and preferred M.O. (*modus operandi*) of direct caring and kind empathy would not have given the person the chance to see if perhaps they longed more for meaning than death.

So, sometimes, the apparently harsh one-liner can be based on concern and compassion. But it should be used only with care and caution.

Another Wake-Up Scenario

I had been working with a couple for almost a year. They had made advances in terms of cooperation, but the wife complained she must be "crazy" since she still felt as if he were cheating on her.

The man requested a private session. When we met alone, without the wife, he told me that yes, indeed he always had been with two women, throughout the entire course of their marriage. I suggested that disclosure would be the best route. In the next session, the wife reiterated her complaint and before my eyes, the man stated, "You must be crazy! I would never do that." Now, a therapist has values as well and human rights, and I do believe therapy ought to be a mutually dignified process (see Ritterman, 1983/2005, pp. 66–84, on Therapy as a Model of Cooperative Exchange). I was not going to be complicit in a lie that would mystify and perpetuate the wife's suffering, nor was I willing to reveal what the husband had told me in private. Here was my zinger: *"Our therapy has now ended. I am no longer able to work with you. I can't explain why. I will do whatever necessary to find you a qualified therapist. But that is no longer me."* They both looked shocked. I smiled sweetly as they gathered their belongings. "No need to pay for the session!" I added. They left my office to convene outside on the walkway. Right then and there, he told her everything. They promptly divorced. I heard that they both did well afterward, and she got married to a man she has loved ever since!

When I used to study the Netter (2006) books of anatomical diagrams of the body, I was most impressed to see the homunculus representation in the brain of the hands and feet. In terms of information received by us humans, we typically get most of it from our hands and feet. In the drawings, they cover the brain. I realized then and there how some aspects of hypnotherapy work with fingers and arm levitations and so forth. When the person is in the correct state, they can take in that information from their hands and feet and generalize it to their entire body. "Ah-ha," I thought, "one image, idea, sensation, or phrase can occupy most of the mind instead of other, destructive images." I realized that even a single memory or sensation can occupy our brain for better or worse and carry much weight. In the negative, an obsessional thought can rule over our lives! In the positive, a single memory can be used to transform a person's experience of him/herself. Tapping the right spot, the right single stroke, may allow helpful memories to come out like scarves from the magician's sleeves. I've described a number of these interventions in a chapter (Ritterman, 2014) called "One-Session Therapy: Fast New Stance Using the Slo-Mo Three-Minute Trance."

(With the Right Stroke) A Tight Space Can Open Creating the Possibility of Change

The well-placed one-line zinger involves simultaneous and sequential multiple landings – they get you coming, going, and where you are. Erickson once asked 29-year-old me my definition of therapy and I said something about changing people. He said, "You change nothing. You create the circumstances under which THEY spontaneously respond and experience a change, no matter how small, positive or negative; and heartened by the possibility of change, go on to make others." First you must create the circumstances for the person to offer you their attention. Then, when they and you are synchronized, sometimes you can introduce or help them find that one image or feeling that can cover their whole experience. We don't remove symptoms or eliminate pain. We facilitate a person's right to pursue happiness. It's a basic human right, and we are part of that as healers.

In Jamaica, I went to the Bob Marley house in an impoverished neighborhood where I was privileged to meet the man called Willing-and-Able who appears in a Marley song. The concrete compound was the place where Marley wrote about the "Three little birds" that pitched by his doorstep singing "Don't worry about a t'ing, cause ev'ry little t'ing gonna be alright." I had an instant connection with Willing-and-Able and told him straight out that the worst thing in my life was my ex-husband who seemed to stand in my way blocking everything I tried to do. His one-line reply helped me change the course of my life. He said: "Your path will widen." And it came to pass.

Great wisdom can be compressed and expressed in a single line or image. In Berkeley, California, there were several terrible episodes of student-on-student violence. Wisely, the school (which is near my home) called in Thich Nich Hahn. I went to see him speak. He said to the students, "When confronted with bitterness and rage, it is like salt. A teaspoon of this salt in a glass of water makes the water undrinkable. But if you put that teaspoon into the river, you can still drink from the river. When confronted with bitterness and rage, become the river."

(A funny version of this occurred when I was pregnant and told an Irish workman in my home, in Philadelphia at the time, that I was miserable to have become so "fat" that I had outgrown all my clothes. With his great brogue he said: "Well, buy them a little biggerrrrr"!)

In my book of poetic meditations, *The Tao of a Woman: 100 Ways to Turn* (Ritterman, 2009, p. 50), I wrote:

> Why try to be
> who you were?
> Didn't you do that already?
> The future doesn't repeat itself.
> This is the time to get acquainted
> with your present self.
> Respond fully
> as you are
> now.

Note

1 The excerpt from Ritterman (2009), *The Tao of a Woman*, is © 2009 by Michele Ritterman. Used with permission.

References

Goldsworthy, A. (2000). *Time*. New York: Harry N. Abrams.

Netter, F.H. (2006). *Atlas of human anatomy* (4th ed.). Philadelphia: Saunders Elsevier.

Riedelsheimer, T. (2001). (Director). *Rivers and tides: Andy Goldsworthy working with time*. DVD: Edinburgh, Scotland: Skyline Productions.

Riedelsheimer, T. (2018). (Director). *Leaning into the wind – Andy Goldsworthy*. DVD. Edinburgh, Scotland: Skyline Productions.

Ritterman, M. (1985). Family context, symptom induction, and therapeutic counterinduction: Breaking the spell of a dysfunctional rapport. In J.K. Zeig (Ed.). *Ericksonian hypnotherapy: Clinical applications* (pp. 49–70). New York: Brunner/ Mazel.

Ritterman, M. (1987, January–February). Torture: The counter-therapy by the state. *Family Therapy Networker, 11*(1), 43–47.

Ritterman, M. (1991). *Hope under siege: Terror and family support in Chile.* (Foreword by Isabelle Allende.). Norwood, NJ: Albex.

Ritterman, M. (2005). *Using hypnosis in family therapy* (2nd ed.). Phoenix, AZ: Zeig, Tucker, & Theisen. (Work originally published 1983.)

Ritterman, M. (2009). *The tao of a woman: 100 ways to turn.* Berkeley, CA: Skipping Stones Editions. (Available in Spanish as *El tao de la mujer.*)

Ritterman, M. (2013). The tao of a woman. In M.F. Hoyt (Ed.). *Therapist stories of inspiration, passion, and renewal: What's love got to do with it?* (pp. 217–231). New York: Routledge.

Ritterman, M. (2014). One-session therapy: Fast new stance using the slo-mo three-minute trance. In M.F. Hoyt & M. Talmon (Eds.). *Capturing the moment: Single-session therapy and walk-in services* (pp. 373–392). Bethel, CT: Crown House Publishing.

Ritterman, M. (in press). Interview: Michele Ritterman, Ph.D. In *The Milton H. Erickson Foundation Newsletter* (M.F. Hoyt, Int.), forthcoming.

CHAPTER 17

Our Clients *Are* Able and Strong
MRI Problem-Solving Brief Therapy in Action
Karin Schlanger and Esther Krohner

"My daughter sent me to see you and, because I am a good mother, I had to do as she asked me to and I requested an appointment. You are highly recommended, but you should know that I have had a lot of therapy in my life!" This is how Catalina, a 59-year-old Chilean woman, introduced her problem in the first session at the Brief Therapy Center of the Mental Research Institute (MRI) in Palo Alto, California. "My daughter believes – and I agree with her – that I am in an abusive relationship. I walk on eggshells around my husband because if I happen to say something that he doesn't like – and I never know what that might be – he yells at me, becomes threatening and abusive. He has never hit me but I am nervous, insecure, and feel vulnerable."

Karin ascertained that Catalina was out of physical danger, at least for the immediate future. Catalina said she had a place to go if she felt threatened, had confided in people around her, and it was clear that when these arguments took place, she felt confident enough to stand up to her husband. Her actions, however, just made the situation more inflammatory and prone to escalation. How does the MRI Problem-Solving Brief Therapy (PSBT) model organize this information and frame the rest of treatment?

When therapists think in an *interactional* way, the focus of treatment is always *the relationship*. Because dangerous behavior for the most part occurs in a context in which people act, react, and respond to what is happening, the client is not just a victim, but also an actor. If the therapist can become curious about the dangerous situation and ask details about the process that culminated in the aggression, both the therapist and the client will be able to construct a new reality around the dreaded incident. People can either be seen as resilient and able to cope or can be seen as victims in need of being put in a protective box, where the only person who has a key is the therapist. The belief in a client's strengths is how the PSBT model *works with the client* to define a problem, chosen by the client to be significant to *them* and that *they* want to change. Working with the client to define the problem is one of the key differences between the PSBT model and many other approaches to therapy.

Another important distinction to point out is that with PSBT a therapist can easily work with one member of the system alone, preferably the person who is the most motivated to change the status quo. Therefore, it will become quite clear that, in Case #1, all the work was done with Catalina. Karin actually never met Henry.

The next significant principle in the model is that of *attempted solutions* (Watzlawick et al., 1974; Fisch et al., 1982). They are defined as communicative actions, thoughts or behaviors performed intentionally and repeated by people within a system of cultural significance. Their intent is to solve a difficulty, but ironically their actions lead them to get stuck: the repeated attempts end up *creating* a problem, perpetuating it and making it worse. When the pattern becomes too painful to the client or someone around them is when a therapist usually gets a phone call requesting help.

Catalina described in great detail that she thought of herself as being a sur- vivor: she had arrived in the US from Chile as a young woman, following her first husband. She had realized soon after having her second daughter that her husband was unfaithful, so she divorced him and relocated to California with her daughters when they were four and six. She supported her family by teaching private music lessons and told Karin she was particularly proud of having been able to afford a house. She had explained that what originally had attracted her to her current husband, Henry, was his sense of humor and his loyalty. She had requested an appointment at MRI because, although her daughter was worried, she knew that Henry would do anything to *keep* this relationship: he felt like a failure because he already had one divorce in his his- tory. He did not want a second.

Near the end of the session, Catalina elaborated:

> I married my current husband, Henry, only five years ago and have lived with him now for seven years. He is not the father of my adult girls because their father was a dead-beat whom I left when they were very little. I have managed my life just fine without Henry, but I didn't want my girls to have to deal with me when I was old. Henry is from the Old Country and when he gets mad he yells loudly and becomes threatening and frightening. I have tried to talk to him at different times, told him to let me know in a calmer voice when I say something he doesn't like. I have even looked at moving out: I went to a real estate office to look at options. After a while that he has been yelling at me, I tell him I am sorry, but I say it in a bad way because I am angry. I just don't want to live this way anymore. I want peace in my life and, ironically, I think he does, too!

Hearing all this story, at the end of the session, Karin said *what*?

> Please go home and prepare two sets of flash cards, one in Spanish and another in Bulgarian (where Henry was originally from) with phrases that

say things like: "I'm sorry, I'm sorry, I'm sorry" and have a drawing of a smiley face on it; another one could say "Maybe next time"; yet another one could say "I love you." If you are feeling creative, you could make one that said something along the lines of, "When you act this way, you really turn me on!'"

Catalina listened carefully, looked intrigued and said: "I think this is going to work!"

What Were We Thinking?

From the point of view of the MRI PSBT model, it is always important to take into account the clients' worldview, *their* reality. In this regard, three important principles influence therapists' thinking. First, Heinz von Foerster's Constructivism (see Watzlawick, 1984): we can only approximate pure and objective truth so, *reality* and *truth* become an *individual construction* because they interact with our context and the relationships we create with it. From this premise, the PSBT approach allows the therapist to believe that the clients are experts in their own lives, and it is therefore the therapist's job to learn the details about what is important to the client. That knowledge then gets incorporated into whatever intervention the therapist will use to steer the client in a different, more productive, less painful direction.

Secondly, Gregory Bateson (1972; Ruesch & Bateson, 1951) in his early work talked about how human beings relate to each other: each action is motivated by the other's response and so on, in an infinite loop of interaction. This way of looking at humans changed the view from an intrapsychic one to a relational one: "A process of differentiation in the norms of individual behavior which results in cumulative interactions among individuals" (Bateson, 1958, p. 175). From this premise flows the therapist's point of view that even in some cases of abuse, while the client might appear to be the one suffering abuse, it happens within the context of a relationship in which there are at least two actors. It is of utmost importance to protect individuals from danger and it is helpful to be able to step back to look at the relationship in order to open the doors to new, more productive interactions, in which the abuse no longer has a role to play.

The final important influence on the work of the MRI Brief Therapy Center is the skillful use of language, ideated by Milton Erickson and promulgated especially by John Weakland. Listening to what words clients use to describe themselves, their realities, and how they see problems gives therapists key insights into how to direct the process of therapy in a useful direction. By definition the contextual frame of a session gives the therapist the role of expert and guide in the process. To promote positive change, it is up to the therapist to pay attention to, and learn, the client's language (what actual words they use to describe themselves, not their mother tongue) and to fit within the client's frame of reference. Therapists have long been taught that if patients – as they are called in conventional models – don't follow the therapist's prescriptions, there must be a resistance to the prescriptions that comes into play. Alternatively, in the PSBT model, resistance occurs when the therapist has moved too fast, neglecting the time and energy to adequately listen for what is important to the client. While these practices may take some time at the beginning of the therapy process, they are well worth the investment, since doing so will allow the communication between the therapist and the client to be more effective when it comes time for the therapist to suggest a different course of action. The client will be able to comply with the suggestions because they will be phrased in a way the client can actually *hear*.

With all of these pieces of the therapy puzzle in place, it is easier to understand that the MRI brief therapist can work with any case that walks in the door. "*You do not need to be a chicken to know when an egg is rotten*," says an Argentinean friend of Karin's. There is little need to become a specialist in any particular issue – alcohol and drugs, gay/lesbian/transgender, family versus individual, cultural sensitivity training, racial equality, phobias, eating disorders, attendance and learning problems, etc. If therapists are willing to listen and have the humility to learn from their clients, the way problems are constructed, de-constructed, and solved is applicable to any system. This represents radical thinking in the 21st century with its growing segregation into specialties and attempts to create protocols and work sheets that put clients in category boxes with labels rather than looking at them as individuals. Although it is ideal to speak a client's native language, it is not imperative if you are willing to listen for cultural differences and allow yourself to be educated. For example, if a therapist tries to convince a Pacific Island family, in any language, that putting grandma into a nursing home is best for everyone, the therapist should not be surprised when the family fails to return for their next appointment: they will not have felt heard and understood. We hope to have made our thinking clear and John Weakland's remark comes to mind (personal communication, 1985) that "Too often we get lost in *explanations* and in so doing we lose track of the *actions* that need to be taken in every particular case in order to promote change."

Catalina returned to her next session, two weeks later. She was smiling broadly and could barely contain her excitement.

Catalina: I was very much looking forward to coming back to tell you how well things have been at home. We have not argued at all! After my last session here I went home and told Henry what you had told me here: that I maybe play a part in our arguments and his getting abusive. You know? His face relaxed! I could see a sense of relief in him that I had never seen before. Since then, he has yelled much less and never has he lost his temper and threatened me. It's been incredible: it's back to when we first met. We are having conversations and our sex life is … well … much improved!

Karin: And did you take the time to make the cards as we had suggested?

Catalina: Yes, I did. I had a great time doing them, but I haven't needed to use them. I guess I'll keep them for a rainy day. When you asked me to make those cards I realized that they were going to say the same things I had been telling him but it was not going to be in the middle of an argument. I was going to be in a better place and that made all the difference.

Karin: I have to admit that I am surprised and a little unnerved by the sudden change, so I suggest that you keep those close because sustainable change happens slowly and with ups and downs.

Karin saw Catalina two more times to make sure that the change was established and durable. She then terminated sessions by leaving the door open, in a typical Brief Therapy Center fashion:

Karin: We agree that our work here is done. If you ever need anything in the future, you know where to find us!

Catalina has continued to send us referrals, which is the best indicator of a satisfied client.

Another Case Example

Professionals using the MRI approach have often endured the criticism that this model can only be used with "uncomplicated" or "light" cases. For this reason, we have picked another, more challenging or "intimidating" (Fisch & Schlanger, 1999) situation to round out this chapter.

Chris was a 15-year-old who had been seen by various therapists in different settings for more than three years to address obsessions/compulsions, suicidal ideation, sleep problems, anxiety, and depression. He was referred to Esther by a psychiatric hospital in the Bay Area where she works in an outpatient clinic. His parents had most recently taken him to the local ER for suicidal ideation and risk of self-harm. The hospitalization was further complicated by the staff having to file a Child Protective Services (CPS) report.

Esther initially met with the whole family. Chris had been trying to manage suicidal ideation for quite some time and had been able to stay out of the hospital, so she inquired: "Are you aware of what contributed to being hospitalized this time? What made it different than the many other times you have had suicidal thoughts?" Chris pointed out that on the day he went to the hospital, he had told his parents about his thoughts and then started banging his head against the wall. In an attempt to restrain him, his father, Tim, had forcibly pulled him to the ground, and eventually both parents brought him to be evaluated at the emergency room. The parents agreed with the basic description of events that Chris had told the therapist. Tim said, "Chris disclosed his thoughts, and he started to bang his head and I stepped in by restraining him while his mom was crying." The parents were mortified that CPS had been called. "CPS criticized us for restraining our son, which was our only option." It is noteworthy that Chris felt very guilty that he had "gotten my parents in trouble, they are really trying their best to help me." All of this was disclosed within the first meeting.

Throughout the description of the events that led to the hospitalization, Chris made statements that his parents had done their best and that he was very sick and out of control. He talked a lot about how depression, obsessions, and compulsions leave him feeling empty and angry. When Esther explored more about what got him angry, he replied by excusing the things that got him angry. For example, "My parents really want me to be social and get great grades, and I see why that is more important to them than having friends and being happier. They want me to have a good education and I am really messing up the investment they have made in sending me to private school, even though I don't like it and people I go to school with use drugs, are mean, and are hard to be around." He also said, "People at school don't want to be friends with me and it is really my fault because I am so anxious in social situations and I get why they would not want me around." Esther noticed the contrast that co-existed between his anger towards his parents and his words to defend their actions.

Chris periodically justified Tim's restraining him, referred to other times his father had used physical force to restrain him and commented about the effect these incidents had on his mother, Diana: "I feel bad that I stress my mom out and that makes her breathe heavy and cry." This attempt to justify and excuse his parents' behavior and take on so much self-depreciation struck the therapist, especially considering that many of his obsessive thoughts surrounded beating one or the other of his parents and harming himself. These interactions shed light on the client's frame of reference and the way he was making sense of his interactions. He was describing himself as being out of control in many areas and therefore undeserving of the things he wanted and hopeless enough that he wanted to disappear. He excused the people who treated him contrary to how he wanted to be treated and in turn used it as further evidence that he was terrible. Esther's interventions were informed by the interactional loop and use of language that was focused on words of protection, effort, guilt and powerlessness.

This case presented a particular challenge because of the life-threatening nature of the problems, yet the MRI PSBT model operates by an "open only one door at a time" premise, which still stood true. Esther spent the first two sessions gathering information from Chris, his parents, and subsequently from his previous therapy providers and psychiatrist. It was clear that the parents were worried and also angry to have their child, to whom they had given everything, threaten them with suicide. To them it was a grand gesture of "*Screw You!*" Diana had a family member who had completed suicide, and Chris sent her into emotional upset when he brought up his thoughts about disappearing.

There were conflicting reactions around Chris' emotions. Diana switched between being angry/spiteful and overly fearful/coddling. Tim had a more unequivocal position on the problem: he interpreted his son's suicidal actions as an offense to him and his wife, and maintained much of the frustrated efforts to "get our son into shape" because Tim himself had suffered from depression and OCD in high school and therefore knew what Chris needed to do to get better. He often expressed his view that "Chris has everything he could possibly need, yet he is suicidal, ditching school, smoking pot and avoiding his responsibilities. He needs more accountability." When the parents were together, Diana would side with Tim, but also send the opposite message immediately after. "No! Chris is very sick and we need to let him work though this stuff, or he might be the kid we read about in the papers who jumped in front of a train."

Chris's report in the first two sessions painted his world as feeling "out of control." He wanted to have fewer outbursts in which he would yell or hit his head against the wall, have fewer tremors and panic, wanted to sleep better and go to school on time. He was willing to stop smoking pot. He said:

> I tried all of the CBT [cognitive-behavioral therapy] interventions. They make me feel even worse. I try to stop my anxious thoughts and the gory obsessive images, but they come back stronger. I try to go to sleep and follow a sleep hygiene routine, but I feel more panicked. I have forced myself to watch the images, and let them be there and apply mindfulness when they come up by tracking the thoughts and noticing them and letting them ride out and paying attention to my breathing [exposure and response prevention therapy], and I have also practiced having the thoughts and images and letting them be there and then using the calming techniques but I feel terrible for having them. I'm a terrible person. My parents are right.

Chris' gory thoughts were about beating his parents or jumping in front of a train or some variant of these two images. He felt extremely guilty and painted a picture of helplessness due to his inability to use the techniques to his advantage. He saw the images as a further indication that he was "bad" and out of control.

In the third session, Chris and his parents agreed that the obsessive thoughts of harm in all its variants were the main problem, and therefore the door was opened to start to promote change. While the parents didn't fully agree about the reason Chris was having suicidal ideation, they both agreed that they did want what was best for him. Because Chris was a client, Esther decided to work mostly with him. Her goal was to build a strong relationship with Chris in preparation for when the parents would be more a part of the therapy and could be more certain they could "commit" to another way of relating to Chris. Also, Esther had a sense that the parents were not being transparent and were withholding information. Chris had mentioned other times when Tim had intervened physically, which the parents had omitted mentioning, as well as reports about Diana's crying fits, which had also been omitted when Esther had inquired about the other times that Chris had threatened/scared them with suicide and how they had handled it. Lastly, because the parents had different frames – Diana saw Chris as more sick and was scared, and Tim was more threatened and angry – Esther wanted to take time to approach this difference and develop language that would enhance their interactional options.

It was also noteworthy that the parents allowed Chris to defend their behavior at his expense (he took on the blame for being out of control even though his mother would be emotionally overwrought and his father would be enraged and pin him on the ground when things escalated). They were an important piece of the interactional structure and their responses to Chris were influencing what he saw as possible. However, Esther needed to get more of Chris's words to use with the parents, so they could have less opportunity to skirt the issues or for Tim to blame and Diana to baby Chris. Esther saw this as the confusing behavior by his parents that was leaving Chris both in control and powerless through his own eyes.

It was clear to both Chris and Esther that Chris harbored contradictory feelings towards his parents: he thought he was spoiled by his parents and at the same time wanted to hit them, which made *him* a bad person. Esther tried to reframe this perception in a way that might be more useful to him: he was managing to pass all of his high-level classes despite missing school and had maintained A grades in a highly competitive prep school. As a part of the reframe, Esther worked with Chris on actions that would still express his anger without having to threaten suicide to his parents. He would accomplish getting their attention in a more positive way. She had worked at establishing credibility with Chris, getting him to feel/understand that she was on his side in fighting this problem. She said:

> These thoughts actually seem to be some sort of protection against actually beating your parents. They seem to be a very creative way to show you are pissed but also staying in control from actually hitting and physically hurting them. Yet they come at the high cost of everyone feeling out of control and quite useless. What if we were to consider that these thoughts and urges have become undeniably *entertaining* to you? You are obviously bored since you can complete all of your schoolwork in a short time and you spend loads of time in bed with these gruesome yet entertaining images. It's like they keep you company! Perhaps you're needing other things to entertain yourself and other ways to deal with what is angering you.

Esther came to this interpretation by comparing and combining the tension between Chris wanting to defend his parents and his seeing himself as terrible as well as him feeling very angry and wanting to get them "off my back." Esther used this intervention, as well, to help lay the tracks for teaching other ways to face what was making him angry as well as to collaborate with his parents on life choices and behavioral choices that he was making. The therapist was trying to level the playing field a bit and create an image (reframe) that made the "out of control" thoughts seem like he could actually control them and that they were a sign of restraint rather than being "out of control."

Chris looked perplexed. He thought, then said:

> I never thought about it that way and you are right – I am very angry at my parents! They say they want me to be happy, but any choice I make they don't like. They push me and threaten me and tease me. They say they want me to share what is going on with me, but I feel very guilty when I admit to feeling depressed or anxious and yes, I am so bored, especially now that I am not returning to my school.

As John Weakland said (personal communication, 1983), "Never drop a winning game," so in the next couple of sessions Esther continued with the approach of looking at the suicidal ideation as an understandable result of being bored and confused and needing more options socially, academically, and communicatively.

As a consequence of the intervention, while the images would still pop up, they were less frequent and less severe. Chris began to see these images as a reminder that he needed to speak up and make some choices about his future. Subsequently, he wanted to spend sessions talking about what he was angry about, and this led to building an interactional picture of how the various symptoms were in some way protecting him and his parents from working through their conflicts around school choices, social choices, substance use and lifestyle choices like exercise and entertainment.

The main difference between the MRI PSBT and the CBT that Chris and his family had experienced previously was that we provided an empowering reframe that the thoughts/feeling were helpful/protective – this made them less disturbing and exposure to them less burdensome, and planted a seed for other ways to protect and advocate for himself. The previous attempted solutions had led Chris and his parents to avoid the suicidal ideation at all costs whereas the PSBT therapist encouraged him to look the suicidal thoughts in the face. The CBT model had talked about exposure but only to drive it away: when the thoughts came, Chris was supposed to relax or in other ways "make them go away." From the PSBT perspective that is a more elaborate way of still avoiding the feelings, which did not work. The avoidance of the thoughts/feelings had become the rut in which Chris was trapped; the new solution used his feelings and thoughts to his advantage as he learned communication skills as well as harnessed his motivation around what he wanted to move toward in his life.

Once the suicidal ideation had subsided, Esther, Chris, Tim, and Diana reconvened and spent multiple sessions talking about how they could "get off Chris' back" so he could figure out what he wanted and so they could figure out what they really wanted for their son. Tim and Diana needed to back off, considerable coaching, and "proof" that their son was willing/able to change. Esther, the parents, and Chris worked on one behavior at a time. The first was figuring out a school option that would allow for Chris to complete the school year. The parents needed help coming to terms with their son not continuing in the high-pressure environment of the school. He was smart, capable, and could potentially return to the higher lanes at a later date, but that for the remainder of the school year it was not a viable option to continue pushing him.

The work became for Chris to use his voice in expressing what was important to him and using his intellect to create options as well as finding things to entertain himself that came at a lower cost than the gruesome images. The work with the parents became giving Chris space and making compromises as well as acknowledging to their son some of the role they played in maintaining the problem. The therapy allowed Chris, Diana, and Tim to mobilize their creativity and find more reasonable ways to influence one another that were less dramatic. Eventually, Chris switched from the highly competitive private school to a public school with an option to start late in the morning, and his sleep improved. Therapy ended when he joined a baseball team and the parents agreed that it was the most important thing for his health since it was something he liked that kept him active and improved his sleep, mood, and sociability.

There has not been any further contact with this family since the decision was made that Chris was so busy with "good" things that it was no longer a necessity to come to therapy.

Conclusion

As seen in the work both with Catalina and with Chris, the MRI PSBT fosters a relationship between the therapist and the client that is flexible, tolerant, sometimes unexpected, and holistic (see Schlanger, 2011, 2013, 2014; Schlanger & Anger-Díaz, 1999). Replacing the fear of sickness or pathology with a search for better problem solving, the therapist can instill hope, creativity, and playfulness into a tense situation, which generates a virtuous cycle propelled by the clients. It is important for the reader to remember, however, that every situation is unique and different, that not every abuse case can be solved with cards, and not every suicidal/OCD situation can be reframed into boredom to promote a different action. We strongly believe that if the therapist chooses to see the clients as able and strong, the message to the client becomes closer to "Yes, we can!"

References

Bateson, G. (1958). *Naven: A survey of the problems suggested by a composite picture of the culture of a New Guinea tribe drawn from three points of view.* Palo Alto, CA: Stanford University Press.

Bateson, G. (1972). *Steps to an ecology of mind.* New York: Ballantine Books.

Fisch, R. & Schlanger, K. (1999). *Brief therapy with intimidating cases: Changing the unchangeable.* San Francisco: Jossey-Bass.

Fisch, R, Weakland, J.H., & Segal, L. (1982). *The tactics of change: Doing therapy briefly.* San Francisco: Jossey-Bass.

Reusch, J., & Bateson, G. (1951). *Communication: The social matrix of psychiatry.* New York: Norton.

Schlanger, K. (2011). Problem-solving brief therapy: The Palo Alto approach to working with a Latino couple. In D. Carson & M. Casado-Kehoe (Eds.). *Case studies in couples therapy* (pp 133–144) New York: Routledge.

Schlanger, K. (2013). Get off your high horse: Reflections of a problem solver in Palo Alto. In M.F. Hoyt (Ed.). *Therapist stories of inspiration, passion and renewal: What's love got to do with it?* (pp. 240–250). New York: Routledge.

Schlanger, K. (2014). Hoy en Palo Alto: Un trabajo en escuelas californianas con población inmigrante. In R. Medina, E. Laso, & E. Hernández (Eds.). *Pensamiento sistémico, nuevas perspectivas y contextos de intervención* (pp. 73–97). Mexico City: Litteris Psicologia.

Schlanger, K., & Anger-Díaz, B. (1999). The brief therapy approach of the Palo Alto group. In D.M. Lawson & F.F. Prevatt (Eds.). *Casebook in family therapy* (pp.146–168). Pacific Grove, CA: Brooks/Cole Publishing.

Watzlawick, P. (Ed.). (1984). *The invented reality: How do we know what we believe we know? (Contributions to constructivism).* New York: Norton.

Watzlawick, P., Weakland, J.H., & Fisch, R. (1974). *Change: Principles of problem formation and problem resolution.* New York: Norton.

CHAPTER 18

Frida Kahlo is Sassy

Clara Haydee Solís Ponce and Pedro Vargas Avalos

The case presented here was informed by the systemic model of the Brief Therapy Center (BTC) of the Mental Research Institute (MRI) in Palo Alto, California (Fisch, Weakland & Segal, 1982; Fisch & Schlanger, 1999; Fisch, Ray & Schlanger, 2009; Weakland, Fisch, Watzlawick, & Bodin, 1974). The therapy took place in a community care program at a university clinic in Mexico City. The community that is served comes from the conurbation of the eastern zone of Mexico City – the population is of low economic resources and low socio-cultural level, with conditions of poverty and urban overcrowding.

Twenty years of teaching and clinical experience have shown us that the systemic model fits perfectly to serve the clinical needs of this population. The therapeutic team was made up of two clinical supervisors and a group of five to ten interns who remained on the team for periods of one to three years, depending on their professional interests. The case was conducted in Spanish in an office with a one-way mirror, and all sessions were recorded in audio and video, which allowed having a digital file recorded on DVD.

There was a reception area where the data for the first contact with the patient was gathered. This information was then passed to the therapist. The interview began with an introduction of the following: the video recording, the presence of the team, the confidentiality of the information, and the time limit. Consent forms were signed. As in the MRI BTC, an initial contract was made for ten regular weekly or biweekly one-hour sessions (Anger-Díaz, Schlanger, Rincon, & Becerra, 2004; Fisch, 1988; Watzlawick, Weakland, & Fisch, 1974; Weakland & Fisch, 1992, 2010).

If there are no doubts or questions about the contract, we usually start the clinical session with the question: *"What is the problem that brings you here today?"* Consistent with the problem resolution model, this is the clearest and most direct way to address the complaint. After that, we ask relationship questions about the context of the complaint. Following the MRI model, the general idea is that the design of the intervention consists of thinking about a behavioral strategy, giving the task, selling the intervention, and monitoring it (Schlanger & Anger-Díaz, 1999). It is assumed that what we seek is mainly a behavioral change. There are cases, however, in which the intervention is designed to modify perceptions about the problem in ways that generate a sense of hope. As Karin Schlanger (personal communication, 2016) has pointed out, having the hope that things will improve is the best incentive to stop unsuccessful attempted solutions. This characteristic is not usually emphasized; it is one of the little-understood elements of the MRI model, and in recent years it has begun to be revalued and emphasized in the practice of brief therapy (Schlanger, 1998; Frusha, Ray, & Hale, 1998).

The Case

Isabel arrived at the university clinic to request clinical psychology services for her nine-year-old daughter, Frida, who was accompanying her. Isabel stated she was a single mother, and that the biological father had not taken care of Frida since Frida was born. The therapist for this case was Clara Solís. To the question "What is the problem that brings her here today?," Isabel responded, "As you can see (as she looked at the girl) I have a handicapped daughter who is now a girl, but soon she will become a teenager and I want to strengthen her self-esteem because she realizes that she is not like all girls." The same question was asked of Frida, and she responded, "In school they bother me, they tell me that I have a stick leg." Frida's left leg had been amputated when she was two years old, so for most of her life she had used a prosthesis that was changed as she grew.

Clara continued to define the problem and explore their attempted solutions. Frida went to an integrated school, which meant that she was not the only girl with special needs there. There were also children from other countries, therefore diversity was natural. At home Frida had obligations and responsibilities like any other girl. Because she was born with a diagnosis of multiple physical malformations, she went regularly to several doctors: an orthopedist, a neurologist, a cardiologist, and a health psychologist.

Socially, Frida was well behaved, intelligent, with a fluent vocabulary and good interpersonal skills. Her mother Isabel had done a good job because her attitude towards her daughter was not to see her as ill, therefore she did not treat her as such. We finished the first session by complimenting both of them for doing a good job and asking them to continue doing more of the same. If the solution is useful, there is no need to modify it.

As discussed in what follows, the case was intimidating for the therapist, and Clara decided to present it to her clinical supervisor, Karin Schlanger, Director of the MRI BTC. Frida's left-leg amputation was complete. There was no stump to support the prosthesis, consequently the prosthesis that was used (which was quite rudimentary) had to be supported with a corset that made Frida's trunk look disproportionate to her body mass. In addition, since the prosthesis was changed as Frida grew, they decided to use a slightly larger size at each new fitting, so that it would last longer. Therefore, whenever the prosthesis was changed, its presence was even more noticeable. In fact, Frida was fitted with a new prosthesis between sessions two and three. Clara oberved that Frida's appearance was noticeably changed, which made the situation more intimidating to her because she could not avoid looking at the prosthesis, either out of curiosity or a morbid sense.

Within the brief problem-solving therapy model, we do not like to talk about "easy" or "difficult" cases, but about "intimidating" cases (Fisch & Schlanger, 1999). This was an intimidating case because the demand seemed legitimate "to raise the self-esteem of Frida" and to teach her at the same time to handle the acts of discrimination that had accompanied her life up until then. The problem-solving brief therapist always thinks of problems and solutions in terms of interactions, and so the next question for Clara was, *"How can I achieve that in actions?"*

Comment. When the case was presented in supervision, Karin's first question was *"Why is the girl in the session?"* Clara answered, "Because the mother asked for it." Karin then asked, *"and why did* she *decide, since you are the therapist?"* Karin's observation suggested Clara's lack of maneuverability in relation to the client because it was Isabel, not Clara, who had decided who was going to be in the session (Fisch, Weakland, & Segal, 1982).

Clara felt intimidated by this family because she did not know how to proceed with the design of therapeutic actions to achieve Isabel's goal. When Karin listened to the presentation of the case, she pointed out something very special: Isabel seemed insensitive and somewhat harsh with the daughter because, although she took care of Frida's medical needs, Isabel did not protect her emotionally. Isabel, presenting her daughter to Clara with "this is my problem," and fixing her eyes on Frida, was not being very maternal. Maybe if Isabel had not made manifest the obvious and did not point to her daughter as someone with multiple physical malformations in a first contact with a group of strangers (the session was in a one-way mirrored office with the team watching), it would not have been perceived as harsh.

The cycle of Isabel's solution attempts can be described as follows: When Frida told her mother that classmates were cruel to her, Isabel told her not to pay attention to them, or to tell the teachers what was happening. Frida did what Isabel advised, but following that advice did not achieve the desired results. While Isabel continued to treat her like a regular girl, she exposed Frida to the schoolyard ridicule, and consequently Frida felt unprotected. That then brought her back to Isabel to ask her mother for help, and there the cycle began again.

Clara's initial asessment changed because of Karin's observation. Following Karin's supervision, Clara's task in the subsequent sessions was to reformulate the goal for which Isabel had come – to go from "raising the self-esteem of Frida" to "being less demanding with my daughter." In other words, to make Isabel the client. In the BTC model, we have a central premise that "each case is, in itself, its own explanation," and for this mother-daughter relationship, reformulation allowed achieving the goals desired by our clients.

Thus, Karin's suggestions for Clara in the subsequent sessions were to spend some time meeting alone with Frida, some time meeting alone with Isabel, and also some time meeting with them conjointly. The intention of seeing Frida alone was two-fold: on one hand, for the therapy team to gain credibility in Isabel's eyes. She brought Frida to be treated because Isabel didn't understand that she was part of the problem; and on the other hand for Frida, so that Clara could generate an empathetic relationship with her, to work with her as a client.

The second session with Frida continued to be intimidating for the therapist. Frida said: "I like psychologists because here I do not have to undress." And when she talked about her problem, Frida said: "In the street people see me. At school my classmates don't let me play, at recess they tell me that I have a stick leg."

Clara: And what do you do when that happens?

Frida: I tell the teacher.

Clara: And what does she do?

Frida: She scolds them and tells them not to say that.

Clara: And what else do you do?

Frida: I tell my mom.

Clara: What does she say?

Frida: Tell the teacher and do not listen to them.

Clara: And that helps you? ...

And the sad little girl said "No." However, she was optimistic and persevering because her right to play was valid. When the relationship with her mother was explored, Frida said that she loved her mother, that she admired her, and that she would like for her mother to touch her more often, and to say to her "I love you." These statements confirmed Karin's hypothesis that Isabel had not been motherly with the daughter.

For the third session Clara continued the interviews with Isabel and with Frida separately. In Clara's session with Isabel, they talked about what she does when Frida tells her about school incidents.

Clara: Frida says that when she complains to you, you say, "Tell the teacher, or do not listen to them."

Isabel: That's right, I do that.

Clara: Well, from now on you are going to stop doing that. Because those comments cannot be ignored, and because accusing the schoolmates has not worked and will not work. We have coached Frida to give intelligent reponses when her schoolmates make those annoying comments, and she says she is willing to try. So, when she complains to you, you will ask her first, how did you handle the situation at that time? And secondly, are you OK? Or, do you need my help to handle this? And, well, if she asks for help, ask her what kind of help, do not assume the answer.

Isabel agreed to cooperate. Clara asked her if she knew about the painter, Frida Kahlo, and she said "No." Then Clara said, "Well, look her up on Google and we will talk about her in the next session."

With Frida, Clara discussed the comments that she received at school that seemed annoying to her. We noted that the way that the situation had been handled up until that point appeared unsuccessful, to which Frida agreed. So, Clara asked if Frida would be willing to do something different, and she said "Yes." Clara explained, "It is not about fighting, it is not about accusing, but it is not possible to ignore." Clara then suggested that Frida give "intelligent responses." At this suggestion, Frida was very interested and excited to hear what it would be to give an intelligent response.

A role-play was then started. Clara acted as a child and began singing the "wooden leg Frida" song that some of the school childen had used to taunt Frida, and Frida was directed to answer: "It's not a wooden leg, it's a prosthesis, and I thought you already knew." Frida understood. Clara said, "Well, let's do it to practice." They did. Clara said, "Well, what does it feel like to give intelligent responses?" She answered "Very good." "Okay, Frida Kahlo, do you think you can put this into practice this week?" and she said, "Of course!"

Clara then asked her if she knew the famous painter "Frida Kahlo," and Frida said, "No."[1] The therapist then took out a book (García-Sanchez, 2004) with the famous paintings by the most recognized Mexican self-portraitist. (After the first session Clara and the team had noted the amazing coincidence that Frida, the client, had the same first name and some similar physical impediments as the famous artist, and the team had suggested bringing some examples of Kahlo's work to possibly share with the client.) Frida immediately showed interest in the book, admired the paintings with keen attention, and listened to the story of how Kahlo was injured, her spine broken, how she was semi-paralyzed and eventually suffered the amputation of a leg. Frida was surprised with the story and the session ended.

Before the next session, Clara went back to consult with the supervisor. Karin suggested to Clara that with Isabel she should first review the effects of the previously assigned tasks, and secondly determine what her main concerns were about her daughter; and that with Frida she should check how she was applying the intelligent responses and determine if she needed help with other areas of her life, as well as continuing to talk about Frida Kahlo the artist.

The fourth session began conjointly, then each was seen separately. Both Frida and Isabel reported changes. They were satisfied with the results obtained when applying the "intelligent responses" idea. The disrespectful, hurtful comments towards Frida had practically disappeared, and Isabel had begun to get closer to her daughter. Both had sought out information about Frida Kahlo and were surprised about what they learned. This filled both of them, particularly Isabel, with enthusiasm and optimism. This example of promoting therapeutic optimism was a kind of "You Said What?" moment in which the girl began to identify with the famous artist who had overcome physical challenges.

In the fourth session, Isabel noted that she was worried about what would become of Frida in life: how she was going to move around the city, whether or not she would have a boyfriend. Little by little, Clara normalized these concerns by suggesting options that could be considered. For example, instead of having the traditional *quinceañera* (15-year-old girl's party), they should buy her a car to facilitate her transportation. She suggested ways that Isabel could begin to treat Frida as a person so that her value as a woman – her skills and abilities, not her physical appearance – were focused on. The message regarding her appearance was to "go slow," because they could find appropriate options once Frida's physical growth was complete. Frida and her mother were advised to look for quality prosthetics, those that were sophisticated, aesthetic, light, comfortable, and especially the kind that are less noticeable.

Being able to consider these optimistic alternative scenarios for the future helped Isabel to soften the relationship with her daughter. Frida, on the other hand, was very happy to think of even more "intelligent responses." Isabel was surprised at how skillful Frida was and how she handled difficult situations, which helped to further improve the relationship between them. The reformulation of the therapeutic objective was being carried out indirectly, because the idea of improving the relationship between them was never presented to Isabel explicitly. This is a clear example of the Ericksonian premise that a small change in one part of the system leads to changes in other parts of the system.

In the fifth session we told Isabel and Frida that the next appointment would be scheduled only after they visited Frida Kahlo and Diego Rivera's *La Casa Azul* in Coyoacán, in the southern part of México City.[2] Isabel agreed to go with Frida.

Treatment Termination

Three months then passed before the sixth session. The team considered this session as a follow-up. During the session Clara asked Isabel whether she had previously known of *La Casa Azul*, and she said she had not. Isabel had carried out the behavioral prescription and the results of the visit were really moving for all of us.

In describing the experience of the visit to the Coyoacán house, Isabel described several things that happened there. To begin with, everyone at the museum saw young Frida walking through the rooms of the house, but the stangers did not look at Frida in the way she had been used to experiencing. Isabel perceived them as looks of surprise and admiration for her daughter – and that made her feel very good.

When continuing the tour, they arrived at Kahlo's studio and saw the renowned painter's wheelchair with her palette on display close by. They were surprised by the objects. Then they moved to the bedroom, and it was there that Isabel and Frida stood motionless (a *You SAW What?* moment!) when they saw Kahlo's prosthetic leg and the special corset on the side of the bed of the most famous and beloved Mexican painter.

From the interview with Isabel:

Clara: … and how did you feel?

Isabel: [*with great emotion*] For the first time, I felt proud of my daughter, and I was reassured to know that my daughter can have a successful life.

Clara: And Frida knows this? Did she hear it from you?

Isabel: No.

Clara: OK, then your next task is to make sure she hears you, tell her more often that you love her, hug her more often and tell her that you are proud of her. I think that will be useful for both.

Isabel expressed willingness to fulfill this task. Frida was also very motivated by the visit and began to show interest in painting. Frida and Isabel were satisfied with the outcomes and the team agreed that therapy could end.

Case Follow-up

An appointment was made for a three-year follow-up interview as part of a research project at our clinic. Isabel and Frida were both present. At that time Frida had just entered high school. When she had only been in classes for a month, the terrible September 19, 2017 earthquake in Mexico City occurred. As a result of the earthquake, Frida's school suffered damage and she had to be relocated to a new high school, one that involved new schoolmates and new teachers.

Despite these sudden changes, Frida responded favorably in this new situation. With respect to the reason for the initial consultation, which was for Isabel "to raise Frida's self-esteem," Isabel said that after the visit to *La Casa Azul*, "Frida began to have very high self-esteem – sometimes she is even a little sassy." This corroborated that the changes achieved had been maintained satisfactorily.

Reflections

The results obtained can be considered as the modification of the failed attempted solutions of Isabel, who saw her daughter as someone with insurmountable limitations who would always need help to get ahead in life. When Frida was nine years old, Isabel began to worry about how Frida would soon enter puberty and would have to face even more difficult situations, for example when her body would begin to develop and she wanted to have a boyfriend. This idea was what was driving her desire for Frida to have a higher self-esteem. That is, Isabel was anticipating a scenario that she perceived as difficult and intimidating. In her daily relationships with her extended family and wider society, Frida had been treated like a regular child; she had domestic responsibilities, looked after her pet, and was schooled as required of any youngster. The social context had, so far, favored an adequate integration of Frida in these different areas. Isabel, however, had neglected nurturing the affective part of their relationship by not giving Frida adequate protection and support.

Isabel's perception and understanding of Frida was changed when she saw Frida's ability to solve her own problems, especially after they visited Frida Kahlo's house. During that pivotal visit, Isabel understood that her daughter, even with her physical limitations, could untimately lead an independent life with a happy and successful future.

Clients' requests for changes in cases where, at first impression, there does not seem to be a way of changing, can be a challenge for a brief therapist. This case shows us, however, that when physical limitations are evident at first impression with the client and the therapist feels it is impossible to offer options, it is important for the therapist to look for additional resources, either conceptual or technical. From this model, derived from the interactional theory of communication of the anthropologist Gregory Bateson (Bateson et al., 1956; Bateson, 2000; Ray, 2007; Watzlawick & Weakland, 1977), no pathological behaviors are seen, but are considered behaviors that may seem anomalous but have a way of fitting into the cultural context in which they occur.

In this case, although at first there seemed to be no options available to satisfy Isabel's request, we applied to ourselves the principle of "going slow" and looking for a perspective that would give us a broader picture to understand the interactional process of the complaint. It also became clear that we needed supervision when we found ourselves at an impasse. Karin's supervision opened options for us to reformulate Isabel's request and thereby promote an implicit optimism that allowed Isabel to have hope for her daughter's future.

Without this reformulation, the work carried out would have represented *more of the same,* just in another version of the already unsuccesful attempted solution. Leaving the mother-and-daugher relationship intact and attempting to have the daughter's self-esteem improve would have been like taking her to the orthopedist for another adjustment of her prosthesis – just something else that needed to be done as part of the handicapped girl's medical follow-up. This small change, working with the reformulation of her objective, allowed Isabel to put aside her attempted solutions (in which she treated her daughter as if she had little expectation that she would get ahead in life). This was enough to start a change in the vision of both the mother and the daughter herself.

In addition, this change of perspective was amplified by using the model of the famous painter Frida Kahlo, and helped Frida feel more comfortable with her physical limitations. The young Frida became capable of seeing her limitations as characteristics that made her really different, but in the sense of a potential that not everyone could have, such as that of a great artist with physical limitations.[3] Our client positively identified with Frida Kahlo. Indeed, when we asked permission to publish this case, our client insisted (and her mother consented) that we use her actual name, Frida.

Notes

1 Frida Kahlo (1907–1954) is considered by some to be a great Mexican artist, political activist, and feminist icon. She began painting, mostly self-portraits, after she was severely injured in a bus accident that required her to use a prosthesis and left her in severe pain for most of her life. Her house, *La Casa Azul*, in Coyoacán, is now a museum and popular tourist attraction. Some of her paintings are displayed there, as are several of the prostheses and braces she wore.

2 *La Casa Azul* (also known as the Frida Kahlo Museum) is the historic house and studio (named for its blue walls) where the famous artist was born, lived, worked, and died.

3 "Feet, what do I need you for when I have wings to fly?" wrote Frida Kahlo (2005, *The Diary of Frida Kahlo: An Intimate Portrait*).

References

Anger-Díaz, B., Schlanger, K., Rincon, C. & Becerra, A. (2004). Problem-solving across cultures: Our Latino experience. *Journal of Systemic Therapies, 23*(4), 11–27.

Bateson, G. (2000). *Steps to an ecology of mind.* Chicago: University of Chicago Press.

Bateson, G., Jackson, D. D., Haley, J., & Weakland, J. (1956). Toward a theory of schizophrenia. *Behavioral Science, 1*(4), 251–264.

Fisch, R. (1988). Training in the brief therapy model. In H. A. Liddle (Ed.). *Handbook of family therapy training and supervision* (pp. 78–92). New York: Guilford.

Fisch, R., & Schlanger, K. (1999). *Brief therapy with intimidating cases: Changing the unchangeable.* San Francisco: Jossey-Bass.

Fisch, R., Ray, W., & Schlanger, K. (Eds.). (2009). *Focused problem resolution—Selected papers of the MRI Brief Therapy Center.* Phoenix, AZ: Zeig, Tucker, & Theisen.

Fisch, R., Weakland, J. H., & Segal, L. (1982). *The tactics of change: Doing therapy briefly.* San Francisco: Jossey-Bass.

Frusha, V., Ray, W., & Hale, D. (1998). The intentional use of implication: An unexplored aspect of the MRI Brief Therapy Model. In W.A. Ray & S. de Shazer (Eds.). *Evolving brief therapies in honor of John H. Weakland* (pp. 57–67). Galena, IL: Geist & Russell.

García-Sanchez, L. (2004). *Frida Kahlo. Colección genios del arte.* México: Susaeta.

Kahlo, F. (2005). *The diary of Frida Kahlo: An intimate portrait.* (Intro. C. Fuentes.) (Bilingual edition.) New York: Abrams.

Ray, W. A. (2007). Bateson's cybernetics: The basis of MRI brief therapy: Prologue. *Kybernetes, 36*(7/8), 859-870.

Schlanger, K., & Anger-Díaz, B. (1999). The brief therapy approach of the Palo Alto Group. In D. M. Lawson & F. F. Prevatt (Eds.). *Casebook in family therapy* (pp. 146–168). Belmont, CA: Wadsworth.

Schlanger, K. (1998). Looking back, looking forward: Reflections in the MRI one-way mirrror. In W.A. Ray & S. de Shazer (Eds.). *Evolving brief therapies in honor of John H. Weakland* (pp. 44–56). Galena, IL: Geist & Russell.

Watzlawick, P., & Weakland, J. H. (Eds.). (1977). *The interactional view.* New York: Norton.

Watzlawick, P., Weakland, J. H., & Fisch, R. (1974). *Change: Principles of problem formation and problem resolution.* New York: Norton.

Weakland, J.H., & Fisch, R. (1992). Brief therapy – MRI style. In S.H. Budman, M.F. Hoyt, & S. Friedman (Eds.). *The first sesson in brief therapy* (pp. 306–323). New York: Guilford Press.

Weakland, J. H., & Fisch, R. (2010). The strategic approach. *Journal of Systemic Therapies, 29*(4), 29–34.

Weakland, J., Fisch, R., Watzlawick, P., & Bodin, A. M. (1974). Brief therapy: Focused problem resolution. *Family Process, 13*(2), 141–168.

CHAPTER 19

Beyond Reason and Insight
The 180-Degree Turn in Therapeutic Interventions

Terry Soo-Hoo

Traditional psychotherapists have long stressed the importance of insight, the key idea being that through insight into one's psychological problems comes the ability to choose more effective behaviors in handling these problems. Historically, the main question has been "Why do you do what you do?" with the answers oftentimes residing within one's problematic childhood.

Unfortunately, there has been limited indication of a solid connection between psychological insight and improving people's abilities to solve their problems. In fact, Jay Haley (1963) suggested that there are times when insight might actually *hinder* therapeutic progress. He proposed that instead of insight, the therapist should focus on generating new, often dramatically unusual behaviors for the client to do. These behaviors will counteract the problem behaviors and thus solve the presenting problem (Haley, 1973). Many of these interventions may be called "paradoxical" strategies (see Fisher et al., 1981; Rosenbaum, 2004; Weeks, 1991). However, I prefer the term "the 180-degree turn" in the way the client approaches the problem (Haley & Hoffman, 1967). Theorists at the Mental Research Institute (MRI) proposed that the more a client tried to solve a problem in a way that does not work, the worse the problem would become (Watzlawick, Weakland, & Fisch, 1974). Furthermore, if this "attempted solution" continued, the very problem that the client was trying to solve would actually be maintained by these ineffective solutions (Weakland, Fisch, Watzlawick, & Bodin, 1971; Fisch, Weakland, & Segal, 1982). In relationships, it is common for people in conflict to engage in such interactional patterns that perpetuate the problem. Family-systems theory uses the terms "circular" or "reciprocal causality" (Gladding, 2002; Becvar & Becvar, 2012). This is the interactional pattern where each person in a conflict is trying to solve the problem by applying pressure on the other person to change. What is needed is not insight into why the clients are engaging in these attempted solutions that do not work, but instead to help them find different solutions that do work and thus break these problematic interactional cycles.

The MRI also proposed that the new solutions must be in a different direction from that of the original, unsuccessful attempted solution (Fisch,

Weakland, & Segal, 1982). Often this is known as "second-order change versus first-order change" (Fraser & Solovey, 2007). "First-order" is change within the same category of solutions, while "second-order" is change to a different category. Sometimes this is also known as "the 180-degree turn in the solution." Although they are called "180-degree turns," this does not mean applying a solution in the exact *opposite* direction of the attempted solution that is not working. Rather, the new solutions are in a significantly *different* direction than the attempted solution. Not all 180-degree turns are paradoxical, but all paradoxical interventions are 180-degree turns. Some therapists take the view that paradoxical strategies should only be used when the straightforward direct types of strategies have failed (Foreman, 1990). Haley (1963, 1976), however, who founded Strategic Therapy, advocated that straightforward approaches, such as cognitive therapy, rely too much on arguing clients out of their illogical problematic thinking and behaviors. Using logic to convince people they should change is difficult when the very nature of the client's problem behavior is based upon illogic. Many problem behaviors are based upon strong emotions that are not related to logic. These emotions stem from perceptions and attributed meanings that have little foundation in reason. Thus, it is often a difficult task to convince a client to change his illogical thinking and behaviors through logical arguments! The question "What is the evidence for your thinking?" works better when the client is able to evaluate his experiences and thoughts in a reasonable and logical manner. If the client says, "I do not have any evidence for the way I think, and I know it does not make sense, but that is just how I feel!" then the therapist is stuck. These are the circumstances wherein paradoxical or 180-degree-turn interventions can be useful alternatives.

A paradoxical intervention can be defined as an intervention that approaches a psychological problem with an unconventional, unexpected twist that is "out of the orthodox" (Watzlawick, Beavin, & Jackson, 1967). Sometimes the case requires innovative or "out of the box" thinking. Paradoxical interventions are effective for a number of reasons. Paradoxical interventions change the rules of the "game" (the interactional pattern). They break up the "rigid thinking and doing" and unbalance the clients so that they have to let go of the attempted solutions to try to regain balance. They also have the effect of breaking the tension in a conflicted relationship. Sometimes the effect is to release pent-up emotions that are beneath the surface. Emotions such as anger, pain, sadness, and anxiety often can be dissipated through paradoxical interventions. However, the goal of a paradoxical intervention is not the release of emotions, but to redirect the energy of the emotions. If a client is successfully directed to engage in a paradoxical intervention that seems outrageous, the client may be distracted from these feelings, thus freeing the client to focus on more constructive and helpful behaviors (Fisher et al., 1981; Rosenbaum, 2004; Weeks, 1991). When interventions are so unexpected and unconventional, they can have a humorous effect. Clients (and sometimes, therapists) often react with laughter to paradoxical interventions. The use of humor in psychotherapy can often be quite paradoxical. In fact, many theorists have discussed the effective use of humor in psychotherapy (see Strean, 1994; Hoyt & Andreas, 2015).

The following are three examples of unconventional therapeutic interventions. Each intervention exemplifies a 180-degree-turn in how the client approaches the problem. They would also be considered paradoxical in nature.

Case Example #1: "Yell More Effectively"

In the following example Mai-Li, a single Chinese-American mother, came to therapy complaining that her 12-year-old son, Brandon, was defiant and oppositional. Her husband had left her for another women four years prior and she was filled with strong emotions, but did not want to talk about these emotions. She complained that her son would not listen to her no matter what she did. She had tried everything to get him to obey her. She had to yell at him just to get him to pay attention. It was obvious to me that the more she yelled at Brandon, the more he resisted. Of course, part of the reason why yelling did not work was that Mai-Li sent very negative, hostile, and demeaning messages to Brandon while she was yelling – such as "You are so lazy!," "You are so stupid, why can't you get A's instead of B's and C's!," and "You are such a failure!" She also conveyed strong negative emotions such as anger and frustration. Furthermore, once she aroused Brandon with these negative messages she was unable to calmly set effective limits. However, even though she admitted that yelling did not work, she said that she could not give it up because if she did not yell at him, he would misbehave even worse and totally ignore her. In fact, Mai-Li reported that her own parents often yelled at her in much the same way.

It can be very difficult for a therapist to challenge such behaviors that have so much history and are being supported by family members around her. My task was to enter "her world" and to work within that unique world. Yelling at her son was a rigid attempted solution to get him to obey – but that was her "frame of reference," which she was not willing to relinquish. Therefore, the therapeutic goal was to make use of Mai-Li's attempted solution in a way that altered the impact of the yelling, which would interrupt the positive feedback loop. However, the intervention had to fit within her cultural context (Soo-Hoo, 1999, 2019).

I initially saw Mai-Li by herself for 50 minutes while Brandon was in the waiting room, and then I saw Brandon by himself for 30 minutes while Mai-Li was in the waiting room. This therapeutic structure was followed for a total of five sessions over a period of six months. Brandon was getting mostly "B's and "C's" in his schoolwork and reported that he was rather bored in school. I got the impression that he was not being challenged academically so he was not motivated to do his best. He had a number of good friends and went to school mainly to be with his friends. He admitted that there were times he did not want to do what his mother wanted him to do at home because she was yelling so much.

Mai-Li reported that she would get really angry when Brandon disobeyed her. It was clear to me that Brandon was reacting to his mother's intense negative emotional outbursts. Mai-Li often appeared frazzled, overwrought, and angry. She was stressed out by her job. She felt her boss was taking advantage of her by overworking her and was underpaying her for all her hard work. Yet, she felt powerless and was reluctant to approach her boss to try to improve her work situation. As a single mother, she often felt overwhelmed by the task of caring for her son by herself, particularly when he disobeyed her.

Mai-Li reported that she saw a therapist previously to get help for her son. However, instead of helping her with her son, the therapist encouraged her to discuss her feelings of being overwhelmed and under too much pressure. He suggested that she must be feeling abandoned and betrayed by her ex-husband and that must make her feel helpless, out of control, and angry. He told her that talking about what was distressing her would help her feel less stressed out, and that she would then be able to deal better with her son. Mai-Li expressed to the therapist that *"In Chinese culture we do not believe in talking about deep troubling feelings."* He also recommended that she should practice relaxation techniques. Her response had been, *"How can I relax when I have so many responsibilities and pressures in my life?"* Consequently, she did not return to him after the one session.

I decided that the focus of the therapy should be mainly on assisting Mai-Li to become calmer and more effective in her parenting with Brandon. However, I also presented two interventions to Bandon to help him disengage from the power struggle with his mother and teacher. He reported that his mother came home from work very stressed out and angry and tended to yell at him a lot. I told him I was helping his mother handle her stress better. The amount of yelling showed how much stress she was under. Would he help me by noticing how much yelling his mother was doing? Together, we made a form listing each day of the week for the next two weeks. He was to mark down the number of times she yelled each day. This type of "observation" task often serves to help a client disengage from the interactional problem pattern. While he was observing and counting the number of times his mother was yelling he was unable to respond with his usual emotional reactions. In addition, he no longer was the problem child, but acting as my "assistant" when he was at home. Furthermore, because he was in charge of the observational task, he could be more in control of the situation.

The second intervention involved a paradoxical injunction. I told him that he appeared to be a "very smart, insightful and sensitive kid" (he demonstrated clear signs of these traits). However, I was worried that if he was to show his mother and teacher how "smart," "insightful," and "sensitive" he really was, they might put pressure on him to do even more than he was doing. He agreed that he did not like pressure. I suggested, therefore, that he should carefully choose who to reveal his real "smartness," insightfulness," and "sensitivity" to, and who not to. He said he wanted to show these things to his uncle who was very nice to him. I also suggested that this type of *"secret"* can be very *"power-ful,"* so he should use it wisely – just as Spiderman's uncle said to Spiderman, *"With great power comes great responsibility."* He recognized this phrase from the Spiderman movies and smiled. He was not entirely sure what this meant but liked the idea of a "secret identity" with special superhero powers.

Thus, I was entering his world. This intervention is an example of the 180-degree turn in the therapy approach. Some therapists might have focused on engaging Brandon to become more cooperative with his mother. However, since his oppositional behavior was rooted in his feelings of being overly con-trolled, he was less likely to respond to direct suggestions to be more coopera-tive with his mother. Instead I gave him an indirect suggestion (in the form of a therapeutic injunction) about how to regain control in his relationship with authority figures such as his mother and teacher. At the same time, this message was designed to activate his strengths. I expected that when he felt "more positive" about himself and "more in control," he would have less need to struggle for control with authority figures. I also met with his teacher and brainstormed with her ways to motivate him and activate his interests in class-room work. However, I explained to her that she needed to present this to him as a "paradoxical challenge." I asked her to tell Brandon the following: *"I noticed you look bored when doing the schoolwork in class. So how about doing some more interesting, yet harder and more challenging schoolwork? Most students your age cannot do this higher-level work, so you probably would not be able to do it either. However, if you would be able to do the 'harder, more 'advanced' work, I and the entire class would be quite shocked and embarrassed that we were so wrong!"* During the next therapy session Brandon reported what the teacher had said. He had looked at an example of the "harder," more "advanced" work and it was more interesting than the regular work. He knew he could do it, and he liked the idea of proving the teacher and his entire class wrong! But he did not want to have the teacher pressure him to work harder. I asked him if he could decide what day he would do the much more difficult, advanced classwork and which days he would ask to do the easier regular class-work everyone else did? This way he might keep everyone guessing about how smart he really was. And, he would be in charge of how much work he would do on any particular day. He liked that idea. I also talked to the teacher on the telephone and asked if she would be flexible about this. She agreed that as long as he did what was required for everyone in the class, she would encourage him to do extra, more advanced work but he could decide how much extra work to do.

One goal with Mai-Li was to help her release some of her stress in a way that would make sense to her and that she could accept. In the process, I wanted to activate her strengths to become more in charge of herself and thus become more effective in her ability to handle Brandon's behavior. I reflected to Mai-Li that I could see that she obviously cared about her son and was working really hard to help him. I told her that we could work together to find a more effective way to help him. I suggested to her that one way to help him would be to develop a "superior" yell. She needed to yell more effectively. "*Show me your best yell,*" I requested. Mai-Li giggled with embarrassment, awkwardness, and hesitation. Some might have interpreted this as she was resisting the idea. However, I understood the giggling as actually the first sign that she was giving up some of the rigidity that was keeping her stuck in the unsuccessful solution. After more discussion and encouragement, she weakly complied with a weak yell. I encouraged her to yell louder – with more energy. "*Try to get in touch with your inner power and strength.*" Then I told her that it sounded like the problem was that her yelling was *too high pitched*. I suggested she try to yell at a *deeper, lower pitch*. I went on to tell Mai-Li that one of the greatest parenting skills is to develop the "*I mean business!*" voice. I pointed out that just as Kung Fu masters spend many years cultivating their special skills, she, as a parent, needed to work hard to develop her special yelling skills. I knew this would resonate with Mai-Li because cultivating *special skills* is a core concept in Chinese culture. Kung Fu masters are the pinnacles of such skills cultivation. They also developed the concept of the "*dantian,*" which is the "chi energy" center of the body. According to Kung Fu masters, to access our true powers, we need to focus on our "*dantian*" and draw our strengths from there. She readily accepted this idea because of her familiarity with Chinese chi energy concepts (Soo-Hoo, 1999). We practiced together how to project a deeper, lower-pitched yell to feel the power inside her, from her *dantian*. Throughout this interaction, she giggled and laughed nervously, but continued to take the practicing seriously. As she giggled and laughed, I could see her releasing anxiety, frustration, and anger. As she became calmer, I directed her to focus on how she was *The Mother* in the family, and she was in charge. At the end of the session, she and I were satisfied that her yell had become sufficiently deep and low pitched. I told her that she was ready to try it out on Brandon.

Also, I advised, when she yelled she should thoughtfully focus on the behaviors she wanted Brandon to stop or change. "*Choose your battles carefully,*" I directed. I asked her to consider what were the most important things she wanted him to do at home. I asked her to try to stop using the global negative messages because those messages were aggravating the situation. I coached her to go slow, take small steps, and to practice her new strategy a little at a time. I also warned her to expect that the new strategy would confuse Brandon, so she might see him act in unexpected ways. It was possible that initially the situation might even get worse. I encouraged her to practice staying "calm" in the face of Brandon's unexpected reactions. I suggested that she would need to experiment with different yells until she found just the right type of yell that would have the best effect. Mai-Li was eager to try this new method on her son, excited in the prospect that at last someone had given her something to do that might work in solving their problems. I could tell that the rationale for the special yelling made sense to her and engendered hope, which would improve her cooperation.

In the session two weeks later, Mai-Li reported that it was awkward at first but after a few tries she had good results. She said that when she yelled in a deeper, low-pitched, in-command voice she was much calmer and more in charge. Additionally, when she yelled in this new way she felt less agitated and angry. Her previous yelling conveyed to Brandon that she was overly emotional, frazzled, and out of control. When she yelled in this more deliberate, conscious, and focused way, she appeared calmer to Brandon and had a renewed sense of being in charge. She also reported that it appeared that Brandon experienced her as less agitated and angry, and subsequently was also calmer and able to listen to her with more attention and focus. Some might say that the "energy" had changed. Mai-Li was instructed to continue to practice developing a superior yell. Over the next few weeks she found she needed to yell less and less. She naturally developed a much calmer *"I mean business!"* voice. Stopping the negative messages was very helpful in reducing Brandon's rebellious behaviors. Focusing on the clear message that "This behavior is not acceptable, and this is how it needs to change" also helped to reduce the conflict. This also helped her gain more confidence in setting effective limits with her son. As Mai-Li presented herself in a more confident, in-charge way, the son reacted more calmly and appropriately. Significantly, as Brandon became less oppositional and defiant, Mai-Li became more positive and nurturing towards him. She began to cook his favorite meals and spent more quality time playing board games with him. These enjoyable times spent with her son also helped to reduce some of the stress from her work.

The next time I saw Brandon he said things were much better at home. His mother was being tougher with him but was much calmer and was yelling much less and actually nicer to him. In the next session, three weeks later, he continued to report that things were getting better at home. He was enjoying school now because schoolwork was much more challenging and interesting. In session four, many weeks later, he said finally his teacher figured out how smart he really was because he was doing the harder, more advanced, classwork every day and getting all "A's" in school. "So, the secret is out!" But that was OK with him. I told him that since the secret was out, as a "smart person" he could now use his "smartness" to figure out how to get along with difficult people. As the power struggle with his mother and teacher dissipated he became much more positively engaged and cooperative with everyone around him.

Mai-Li also continued to improve over a period of months. She was able to learn principles, or concepts, such as "I am in charge at home when I am calm, clear and focused," "Limits are most effective when I am firm but fair," and "I can teach respect by modeling respect for my son." These principles and concepts could generalize to other aspects of the client's life. In this case, Mai-Li was able to tell her boss that she felt he was unappreciative of her hard work. She asked for a raise in her salary, pointing out that she was an important asset to the company. So far, she had worked hard to contribute to the company and would contribute even more with a raise. She was calm, confident, and assertive, but *respectful*. Her boss noted that lately she appeared much more confident, focused, and efficient in her work and granted her the raise!

How did I know that Mai-Li would be open to this intervention? She mentioned that she enjoyed Kung Fu movies and read a lot of Kung Fu novels as a child in Hong Kong. So, the concept of chi energy and inner power was part of her worldview. She was searching for a way to regain a sense of control in her relationship with her son. Her family used yelling as a way to assert authority and control. However, this method was not working with her son and, in fact, was aggravating the problem. My goal was to develop a "frame" that would help her feel more in charge of herself in response to her son's inappropriate behavior. "Yelling more effectively" became a metaphor for regaining her power and control, which fit her cultural context.

Case Example #2: "The Jumping Superstars"

This example deals with a very common classroom problem that often challenges even experienced teachers. A school psychologist at an inner-city school contacted me wanting my assistance with a problem child. Ten-year-old Jonathan was "driving the teacher crazy" in the classroom and the school psychologist was unable to help the teacher find an effective solution to the problem. I agreed to meet with Lisa, the fifth-grade teacher, to explore the problem and to offer any assistance I could. Lisa was extremely exasperated with Jonathan's disruptive behavior. She reported that Jonathan would make funny noises and say outrageous things in class. For example, he would make strange, inappropriate noises in class and other students would laugh. Lisa would reprimand him by telling him he was a "bad boy" and needed to stop making inappropriate noises. As soon as she turned around, Jonathan would yell out "Piggy Oink, Oink!" Unfortunately, this resulted in the entire class laughing even louder. This behavior would seriously upset Lisa, and she would send him to the principal's office, which had no effect on changing his inappropriate behavior. Other times, she would make him sit in the corner by himself as punishment. He would continue to make inappropriate funny noises while sitting in the corner. Using punishment only escalated his problem behaviors. Lisa called Jonathan's mother to report how Jonathan was acting inappropriately in class. However, Jonathan's mother was puzzled because he was fine at home and she did not understand why Lisa could not correct his misbehavior at school. The school psychologist suggested Lisa try a reward schedule. If Jonathan was able to reduce his disruptive behavior to two per day he would get a reward, and if the disruptive behaviors totaled less than ten at the end of the week he would get a bigger reward. This also failed to improve the situation.

Consultations with schools can be challenging because such consultations involve understanding how a teacher has been handling a problem as well as understanding the child with the presenting problem and knowing what has already been tried by the school psychologist. Furthermore, new interventions must fit within the classroom as well as the school system (Soo-Hoo, 1998). I agreed to visit the classroom to observe Jonathan. After observing Jonathan in the classroom, I offered Lisa a reframe, or different interpretation, of the situation. I suggested that although Jonathan was getting a lot of negative attention through his behaviors, I thought that in fact he wanted "positive attention" but did not know how to get it appropriately. Lisa readily agreed with my assessment but believed she did not know how to help him. I first validated Lisa, based on my observations and my interview with her, for being a very caring and devoted teacher. I speculated that whereas some teachers would try to get rid of a problem child like Jonathan and refer him to a special day class for children with behavioral problems, she was committed to helping him overcome his problems. Lisa agreed that there were times when Jonathan could be a *good kid* when he was not being a *class clown*. She felt bad about not having been successful in helping him so far. I suggested that a good first step would be for her to try to spot positive appropriate behaviors and give Jonathan a lot of praise and positive attention.

In addition, I advised Lisa that it would be helpful for her to do something that would disrupt the undesirable interactional problem cycle that had developed. Lisa was instructed to tell Jonathan that she saw that he had a lot of pent-up "energy" inside. She was to explain to him that these energies were causing him to behave (act out) in ways that were interfering with his ability to concentrate and focus on his schoolwork. She was to tell him that many people in the school had seen that he was a "smart boy" who could do a lot of "good stuff," but these pent-up energies were getting in his way. She was to let him know that the whole school wanted to help him do his best and be successful. Lisa was to explain to him that the school had developed a way to help him and, in fact, also "help the entire class" release these energies in a productive and healthy manner. Lisa told Jonathan that "Tomorrow morning I will explain to the entire class about an important exercise we are going to be doing":

> Starting tomorrow every morning the class will engage in a healthy exercise called "Jumping Superstars." Each day everyone builds up pent-up energies. These energies can cause frustration and disruptive behaviors that can carry over from one day to the next. We need to release these energies in a healthy way. We are going to practice releasing these energies in class as the first thing we do in the morning. So, we are going to become "Jumping Superstars." Basketball players use this exercise to develop their jumping skills. This helps them become more focused and play better. (Lisa would demonstrate how to jump in place.) We are going to jump in an easy relaxed way. The goal is to release tension in our bodies. As each person jumps, he or she will think of releasing unwanted energies. While we are jumping we will release the energy by saying the sound "Ahh!" as we land after each jump.

She further explained:

> Students should not say inappropriate words as they jump. This will help everyone feel better and focus on classwork better. If anyone begins to say or do inappropriate behaviors during the rest of the day, it is a sign that the person did not do enough jumping in the morning. So that person will need to go to the corner to jump some more to release the pent-up energies. If a child says that he or she is tired and does not want to jump anymore, the teacher will say that he or she could rest. But if the energies returned he would need to jump some more to release them.

Also, I had cautioned Lisa to be sure that everyone in the class could do the jumping exercise without feeling overly stressed, and she had to be sure there were no medical issues to consider. If someone could not jump in place, he or she could jog (run) in place, which would be less physically difficult. Lisa thought everyone would be able to do the jumping in place but promised to monitor their performance to be sure they were not overly stressed.

The next morning, Lisa presented this new activity to the class as a new way of helping everyone in a caring way instead of punishing anyone for bad behaviors.

Initially everyone in the class felt awkward, silly, and embarrassed while trying to jump in place. However, very quickly this became a routine that everyone enjoyed. It was fun and had an important purpose. In fact, there was a significant calming effect on the entire class. Students seemed more focused on their classwork with less restlessness, excessive talking, and disruptions. This simple exercise had a significant calming effect on Jonathan. In fact, it was discovered that jumping two times a day produced even more positive effects for the entire class. Very quickly he was no longer the "class clown" that got attention by provoking other students to laugh at him. Since the message was that all students had energies that needed to be released, he was now just like everyone else in the class. Furthermore, as a reward for doing so well so quickly he was designated as a member of the "Jumping Superstar Leaders"! He along with two other students, who also had "too much energy," were asked to lead the entire class in the jumping exercises twice a day. In addition, the "Jumping Superstar Leaders" would help Lisa identify when someone was showing signs of too much energy in class and therefore needed to do more jumping. This further changed his role from the problem child to the class helper and leader! Jonathan's inappropriate behaviors dramatically dissipated, and he became a respected class leader. Remarkably he was observed reassuring two new students who were showing signs of anxiety and nervousness about starting a new school and adjusting to a new classroom. He told them everyone had pent-up energies, but he would teach them how to jump to release these energies and that would help them feel better!

As can be seen, the intervention takes a 180-degree turn from the attempted solutions that had failed. The focus moved away from trying to suppress Jonathan's inappropriate behaviors to releasing and redirecting the underlying energy that was driving the inappropriate behaviors. There is also an element of a "strength-based" approach (Soo-Hoo, 2018). The intervention created a new "frame" of helping the client to "do better" because people recognized his strengths and positive attributes. This was in contrast to punishing him for "bad" behaviors because he was a "bad boy." Furthermore, there was special power in depathologizing his behavior by involving the entire class in the intervention. In my experience class clowns have a desperate need to be accepted and to belong. The "strengths-based" approach also focused on changing the child's role from that of the "problem child" to a respected member of the class that could be a helper and leader.

Case Example #3: "Kiss My Ass"

In this example, I realized that a previous therapist had taken a fairly direct approach that did not work. Accordingly, from the MRI perspective it was natural for me to take a 180-degree turn in approaching the problem. Mandy, a 26-year-old woman, came to therapy complaining that Josh, her 27-year-old husband of five years, constantly bickered with her about small things. He was upset that she did not have dinner ready on time when he got home, she did not keep the house clean and orderly enough, and did not wash his clothes just right, etc. She had tried her best but thought that his standards were too high and that he was too rigid. He reportedly obsessed on small things that were not that important. He constantly told her how his mother would do the jobs much better! She tried to defend herself, but that only led to more arguing and fighting. Then, she got frustrated and angry and attacked him for being a "control freak" and a "Momma's boy"! She also suspected that he had been getting more irritable because of his problems at work and was taking out his frustrations on her when he got home. She reported that their sex life had been very satisfying when they were not fighting. However, because of the increase in fighting, sex was becoming almost non-existent. She was quite distressed about this.

The couple initially went to a therapist who focused on the unresolved issues between the husband and his mother. This therapist suggested that since Josh was spending so much time in his mother's house, he obviously had unresolved attachment issues. He was overly enmeshed with his mother. The therapist told them that he needed to individuate and separate more cleanly and thoroughly from his mother. He should develop clearer boundaries with her. The previous therapist had also reportedly stated that Mandy had "unresolved family issues at the point of departure from her family of origin." In addition, the therapist had also tried to improve their communication skills. She suggested that the couple try to express their emotions in a more direct manner by using *I statements* such as "I feel angry when you compare me to your mother." However, their attempts to communicate more openly only fueled the conflict. Both Josh and Mandy thought that the previous therapist did not really understand them and was not very helpful. They terminated therapy after four sessions. Since Josh felt that the previous therapist took Mandy's side and blamed him for the problems in the relationship, he refused to come to therapy with Mandy this time.

This interactional pattern is quite typical. Josh criticized Mandy for inadequately handling her job as wife. She tried to defend herself by telling Josh that she was doing the best she could, and that his standards were too high. This implied it was his problem. Josh escalated his complaints that his mother had even higher standards. So, in Josh's eyes, there must be something wrong with Mandy. Much of their relationship was focused on how each person was trying to convince the other that they were right and the other was wrong and therefore, needed to change. "All my friends agree with me – you are the odd one with the problem!"

They also expressed illogical assumptions, such as "If you really loved me you would agree with me and do what I want!" or an even more outrageous message, "If you really loved me you would behave like my mother!" Clearly these illogical assumptions can be challenged, and some clients might benefit from such challenges. However, both Mandy and Josh had difficulty logically and reasonably examining and evaluating these assumptions. For clients such as these it is more effective to engage them to behave in ways that break up these ineffective problematic interactional patterns (Soo-Hoo, 2005).

The first task was to reduce the emotional reactivity of both of them. However, since only Mandy was coming to therapy we needed to focus on how she could lower her reactivity, which would then hopefully lower Josh's reactivity. To do this I explored her strengths and helped her to be calmer in response to her husband's criticism. Mandy explained that what really enraged her was when Josh compared her to his mother. The message she got was that she was a bad wife because she was not as good as his mother. "If he thinks his mother is such great stuff, he should marry his mother!" I empathized with her emotional reactions and acknowledged that feeling angry and hurt are natural reactions to what he said. However, I asked about what good things there were in the relationship that would be worth saving. She acknowledged that except for these fights the relationship was actually quite good. During those good times, they shared a lot in common and really enjoyed each other's company. They shared the same sense of humor. I observed that there was still enormous love and affection in the relationship, and she readily agreed. We established that the focus of the therapy would be on reducing these fights and to reactivate all the positive things in the relationship.

Since Mandy said Josh was under stress at work, I asked her would there be a way she could help him relieve some of the stress when he came home? She became rather resentful of the idea that she had to help him, because he had been mistreating her. This initial strategy was to try to engage Mandy to initiate more mutual support for each other at home. It was evident that she was too angry with Josh to think of supporting him in his time of stress.

Interventions have to make sense to the client. They have to fit a frame of reference that has the right meaning. Since Mandy was angry and resentful at Josh, my goal was to focus these emotions in a more productive way. I suggested that it sounded like she wanted to stand up to his unfair mistreatment of her. If that was the case, then she needed to find a way to send this message to him that did not lead to more fighting! Would there be a "dramatic" way to send the message that she was not going to put up with his "unreasonable," "unfair," and "mean" (her words) criticisms of her? The 180-degree turn is moving away from the attempted solution that is not working, in this case moving away from defending herself and arguing with her husband about who is right (Soo-Hoo, 2005).

After much discussion we decided that the next time Josh criticized her, she would truly show him what she thought of his criticism. She would act out the message in a dramatic way. I suggested that the next time he unjustly criticized her, she should turn her backside to him, lift her skirt, bend over and shake her butt at him, and if she was especially angry with Josh she could add "Kiss my ass!" She laughed and thought the idea was hilarious! However, she was worried that once he started to criticize her, she would become so angry that she would not have enough self-control to do this. I suggested that perhaps she needed to first practice this when she was not angry. What if she was able to find a time when both of them were not fighting? She would ask Josh to sit down while she remained standing. I said, "Calmly say to him, 'I want to make a statement about how I feel about the way you have been *mean* to me. This is what I think of how you have been *mean* to me!" Then, I repeated, "Turn your backside to him, lift your skirt, bend over and shake your butt at him!" If she felt really bold and *sassy* she should add, "Kiss my juicy ass!" Mandy laughed with glee at the prospect of such an outrageous act of *defiance*! She was excited at the prospect of waving her ass at him. This was the perfect message. She left the office with a big grin on her face.

Mandy returned in three weeks and said, "Amazingly, each time I did this, both of us broke out in laughter and then had great sex!" She also discovered that this strategy worked even better when she decided not to wear underwear! In fact, they were having much more sex during the last three weeks than they had for a long time. It really worked. When Josh criticized her for not doing a good job cleaning the house, she just waved her butt at him. He laughed and got the message. It had become a fun game they played to reduce some of the tension between them. It also seemed to be a good way to help Josh release some of his work-related stress. Mandy also reported that one time, when Josh criticized her saying that his mother could do a better job at cleaning the house, she responded by lifting her skirt and waving her butt at him and asking, "Can your mother do this?" From then on, he did not bring his mother up again.

Once the fighting dissipated, Mandy said they were able to become more emotionally open with each other again. Mandy told Josh that the first session with me was very helpful and asked him to come with her to the next one. Josh agreed to come with her to couple therapy. Therapy with both partners progressed to working out other important issues in their relationship. With significant reduction in anger and hostility they were much more open to acknowledging how much they loved each other and vowed to show more appreciation. Josh agreed to help out more to keep the house clean and Mandy agreed to be more supportive of Josh and acknowledged how hard he worked during the day. Josh also conceded that he needed to focus more attention on his own marriage and spend less time at his mother's house. This was especially true since now he had renewed positive reasons to look forward to going home to see Mandy! Therapy successfully terminated after five sessions.

There are many reasons for the success of this therapeutic intervention. I activated Mandy's strengths, which allowed her to be calmer and more confident in approaching Josh. She was able to use the homework activity to disengage from the interactional pattern that was not working for them. In the process, she was able to replace the ineffective interactional pattern with something that worked much better. One might notice that there was an element of "provocative humor" in the intervention. Instead of confronting her husband about how he was wrong, unreasonable, a "control freak" and therefore he needed to change, she performed an outrageous behavior that provoked laughter from him. She was standing up to him in a humorous way that did not say he was "bad" or "wrong." Yet at the same time Mandy's behavior had a clear sexual message that Josh could not ignore. To her credit she performed this outrageous yet humorous gesture in a way that made it safe for Josh to approach her sexually.

How did I know that Mandy would be open to such an intervention? She showed signs of having a good sense of humor and she said that she and Josh shared a similar sense of humor. She reminisced that they used to have more fun and laughed together more often. Furthermore, the couple had great sex when they were not fighting. So, part of the strategy was to generate an intervention that would make use of these strengths and positive attributes.

The goal was to help each of them get on with their lives. When the couple was able to interrupt the problematic cycle and move closer together, they became much more focused on how to sustain the positive aspects of their relationship. As each person stopped criticizing and attacking the other, they were freer to share their positive feelings. Through mutual support and enjoyment of each other, there was a natural maturing and growth of each individual within the relationship.

Conclusion

The previous examples highlight some of the principles of the 180-degree turn in MRI therapeutic strategies. Each case was unique and therefore therapeutic strategies had to be tailored to fit the unique circumstances of each clinical situation. The common element in all three examples involved thinking "outside the box." It is important for a therapist to recognize when certain strategies did not or will not work. The task is then to be creative and innovative in generating the critical 180-degree turn in the solution. Another important point in these examples involved activating the clients' strengths, which allowed the clients to feel more empowered and, therefore, more capable to carry out the interventions. Furthermore, using the clients' strengths enhanced the therapeutic alliance and established more credibility for the therapist. These two factors increased the likelihood of the clients complying with the therapeutic interventions. Finally, a critical element of any therapeutic intervention is the process of entering the client's unique world and to be able to work within that unique world. Interventions need to fit within the cultural context of the client. Ultimately, no matter how brilliant the intervention, it is quite useless unless the client agrees to implement it.

References

Becvar, D. S. & Becvar, R. J. (2012). *Family therapy: A systemic integration* (8th ed.). Boston: Allyn & Bacon.

Fisch, R., Weakland, J.H., & Segal, L. (1982). *The tactics of change: Doing therapy briefly.* San Francisco: Jossey-Bass.

Fisher, L., Anderson, A., & Jones, J.E. (1981). Types of paradoxical interventions and indications/counterindications for use in clinical practice. *Family Process, 20*(1), 25–35.

Foreman, D. M. (1990). The ethical use of paradoxical interventions in psychotherapy. *Journal of Medical Ethics, 16*(4), 200–205.

Fraser, J.S., & Solovey, A.D. (2007). *Second-order change in psychotherapy: The golden thread that unifies effective treatments.* Washington, DC: APA Books.

Gladding, S. T. (2002). *Family therapy: History, theory, and practice.* Columbus, OH: Merrill Prentice Hall.

Haley, J. (1963). *Strategies of psychotherapy.* New York: Grune & Stratton.

Haley, J. (1973). *Uncommon therapy: The psychiatric techniques of Milton H. Erickson, M.D.* New York: Norton.

Haley, J. (1976). *Problem-solving therapy: New strategies for effective family therapy.* San Francisco: Jossey-Bass.

Haley, J., & Hoffman, L. (1967). *Techniques of family therapy.* New York: Basic Books.

Hoyt, M.F., & Andreas, S. (2015). Humor in brief therapy: A dialogue. *Journal of Systemic Therapies, 34*(3), 13–24; and *34*(4), 54–60.

Rosenbaum, R.L. (2004). Paradox as epistemological jump. *Family Process, 21*(1), 85–90.

Soo-Hoo, T. (1998). Applying frame of reference and reframing techniques to improve school consultation in multicultural settings. *Journal of Educational and Psychological Consultation, 9*(4), 325–345.

Soo-Hoo, T. (1999). Brief strategic family therapy with Chinese Americans. *American Journal of Family Therapy, 27*, 163–179.

Soo-Hoo, T. (2005). Transforming power struggles through shifts in perception in marital therapy. *Journal of Family Psychotherapy, 15*(3), 19–38.

Soo-Hoo, T. (2018). Working within the client's cultural context in single-session therapy. In M.F. Hoyt, M. Bobele, A. Slive, J. Young, & M. Talmon (Eds.). *Single-session therapy by walk-in or appointment: Administrative, clinical, and supervisory aspects of one-at-a-time services* (pp. 186–201). New York: Routledge.

Soo-Hoo, T. (2019). Asian Americans in couple and family therapy. In J. Lebow, A. Chambers, & D. C. Breunlin (Eds.). *Encyclopedia of couple and family therapy* (pp. 1–7). New York: Springer Publishing.

Strean, H. S. (Ed.). (1994). *The use of humor in psychotherapy*. Lanham, MD: Jason Aronson.

Watzlawick, P., Beavin, J. H., & Jackson, D. D. (1967). *Pragmatics of human communication: A study of interactional patterns, pathologies, and paradoxes*. New York: Norton.

Watzlawick, P., Weakland, J.H., & Fisch, R. (1974). *Change: Principles of problem formation and problem resolution*. New York: Norton.

Weakland, J. H., Fisch, R., Watzlawick, P., & Bodin, A. M. (1971). Brief therapy: Focused problem resolution. *Family Process, 13*(2), 141–168.

Weeks, G.R. (Ed.). (1991). *Promoting change through paradoxical therapy*. New York: Brunner/Mazel.

CHAPTER 20

They Said *What?*
Themes and Lessons
Michael F. Hoyt and Monte Bobele

The contributors have provided fascinating stories and clinical discussions based on their various theoretical orientations. Before considering particular issues, we offer this general description of a *You Said What?* response:

> Hearing about a statement, action, or directive that is far enough from a listener's expectation or usual way of operating that the listener thinks, or even says aloud, *"You Said What?"* (or some variant thereof, e.g., *"Wow – how'd you think of that!"* or *"Far out!"* or *"Really – what happened?"*).

Readers all bring with them different expectations and experience levels. Some are clinicians with many years of experience with creative, unconventional interventions; for others, all of these *You Said What?* moments are new and may seem unusual and provocative. As I (MB) recounted in Chapter 4, early in my professional training I attended a weekend workshop that turned out to be a long and wonderful *You Said What?* experience that opened my eyes to many different ways of working successfully with clients.

Some of the chapter authors' descriptions are original, whereas others are derivations of practices once novel, but now more well-known to most therapists. Some *"You Said What?"* interventions may seem shocking, or even outrageous, especially to newer therapists; some disrupt unsuccessful solutions while seeming less extreme; others may appear to come out of nowhere. What they all have in common is that they surprise the reader – and often, the client. All of our contributors intended to introduce new experiences and meanings beyond well-worn, more-of-the-same, approaches. Just as when a client says, "That's a really good question," meaning "It makes me stretch beyond and outside the way I was thinking," readers may have a *You Said What?* moment when the intervention seems counterintuitive or when it dramatically challenges what they might have considered doing in such a situation. *You Said What?* interventions invite a significant shift in perspective.[1]

Clients frequently arrive at a therapist's doorstep after a long struggle with attempted solutions to problems that haven't worked. They may benefit from a new way of thinking about themselves, their problems, their abilities, their relationships, and their options. These can lead to a new way of behaving. Sometimes a therapist's respectful listening, simple skill instruction, and logical problem-solving will do the trick, but many times, that is not enough. When previous solution attempts have failed, "second-order" change (Watzlawick et al., 1974; Fraser & Solovey, 2007) is needed. Consider these *You Said What?* examples from the preceding chapters:

- A woman who had been a victim of group satanic abuse sought help for her emotions. Rather than allowing her to continue her pattern of now avoiding groups, the therapist invited her to participate in therapy with a witnessing group! At first, she was very distressed by the idea of a group and balked, but ultimately found the witnessing group healing (Duvall, Chapter 6).
- A mother and her daughter, who had had a leg amputated, came to therapy and didn't have the hope that someone with one leg could be successful. The therapist directed the mother to be more supportive and less critical of the daughter, and then introduced them to the story and work of one of the country's most famous artists. They discovered that she, too, had only one leg (and happened to have the same first name as the daughter!). The mother later explained (with great emotion), "For the first time, I felt proud of my daughter, and I was reassured to know that my daughter can have a successful life" (Solís and Vargas, Chapter 18).
- A suspicious man was given the assignment of looking for and reporting confirmatory evidence that others were threatening him. He returned, admitted that he could not find any such evidence, and began to shift his view of others and himself (Cannistrá, Chapter 5).
- An agitated and belligerent man in the emergency room became sympathetic and calm when the consulting therapist appeared in a wheelchair (Hoyt, Chapter 10); similarly, in Chapter 4 Bobele presents a transcription of Harry Goolishian working with a client whose desire to donate his post-suicide body to medical science gave way to the client's concerns about the seemingly inept therapist.
- A man in couple therapy claiming to be calm, cool, and collected was asked "Would you like to know more about yourself?" and then, switching channels to the body, was guided to notice the contradictory physical evidence of his clenched, angry hands[2] (Ritterman, Chapter 16).
- A bereaved woman angry at the person she believed responsible for the death of her baby was told that she would be letting the person "off easy" if she killed her (Bobele, Chapter 4).

Different Theoretical Approaches Can All Produce "*You Said What?*" Interventions

We all tend to look through our particular "lenses" (Hoffman, 1990). Therapists of divergent theoretical orientations, of course, could cast a particular *You*

Said What? intervention in terms of their own preferred conceptualizations. Directing clients to perform their symptoms might, in a strategic therapy framework, be seen as a paradoxical strategy designed to disrupt unsuccessful avoidance and change interactional patterns; whereas in a Dialectical Behavior Therapy (DBT: Linehan, 1993) or CBT framework it might be seen as engaging in "opposite action" that either teaches stress tolerance and/or serves as a desensitizing form of "exposure and response prevention" (Rowa, Anthony, & Swinsen, 2007). Imagine someone observing a two-chair Gestalt therapy process such as "Imagine your father in that chair and talk with him." A psychodynamic therapist might see "transference" being enacted; a redecision therapist might ask, "Who's been living in your head?"; cognitively oriented therapists might describe the same clinical interaction in terms of "maladaptive self-schemas"; a narrative therapist might talk about "personification" and "externalization" and wonder aloud if these are the client's preferences and how she was "recruited" (indoctrinated, brainwashed) into particular beliefs; a solution-focused therapist might understand the second-chair persona as an "exception" to the problem; an Ericksonian might focus on the hypnotic suggestion of a new experience; and an MRI therapist might conceptualize the process as the evocation of second-order change via the disruption of a positive feedback loop in an unsuccessfully attempted solution!

The term "paradoxical intention," which is often associated with strategic approaches, was originally introduced in 1947 by the existential logotherapist Victor Frankl (1991).[3] Alfred Adler (see Ansbacher & Ansbacher, 1956) talked of waving a "magic wand" long before Steve de Shazer (1988) asked "The Miracle Question." In a conversation about EMDR (Levin, Shapiro, & Weakland, 1996), the originator, Francine Shapiro, emphasized intrapsychic "reprocessing" aspects of the procedure, whereas MRI's John Weakland highlighted the current interpersonal context -- and they both agreed that the therapeutic relationship was important and that it was seldom enough to look for a single factor. All of which is to say: *How one looks influences what one sees* (Hoyt, 2000, 2017). It's complicated, but important not to confuse our words and theories with what actions may be occurring.[4]

Characteristics of *"You Said What?"* Interventions

"What makes zingers zing?" Michele Ritterman asked in Chapter 16. *You Said What?* moments are surprising and therapeutically effective. We see a number of active ingredients. Together they promote a *You Said What?* experience.

Respect and Empathy.[5] Ritterman noted that "the well-placed one-line zinger involves simultaneous and sequential multiple landings – they get you coming, going, and where you are." *You Said What?* moments involve appreciating clients' worldviews, as Andy Austin (Chapter 2) did with his client's image of her children being separate from her cocaine use; as Bobele (Chapter 4) illustrated when he convinced a woman wanting revenge that her intended victim will suffer more if the woman refrained from committing assault; as Shelley

Green (Chapter 9) modelled with a couple who believed in reincarnation and that the husband and the woman he was having an open affair with had been twins in a previous lifetime; as Joe Goldfield (Chapter 8) achieved with an angry man who was feeling stressed-out and disrespected; as Ritterman showed in her work with a Catholic woman feeling guilt about having an abortion; as Flavio Cannistrá (Chapter 5) managed when he acknowledged that life had been very "shitty" for his client and apologized for suggesting that all the client's miseries could be resolved briefly; and as Chris Iveson (Chapter 12) actualized as he conducted conjoint solution-focused therapy with a man and his imaginary/hallucinatory girlfriend (!). In each case, speaking the client's language – using his or her images, metaphors, and prosody – facilitated the connection.[6] In Chapter 14, David Keith pointed out that his practice of "therapeutic teasing" actually conveys affection and respect by suggesting to his clients, "I care about you and you're smart enough to grasp that I am being playful."[7]

Surprising and Attention-Grabbing. A characteristic of effective brief therapies that extends over multiple theoretical approaches is the *introduction of novelty* (Budman, Hoyt, & Friedman, 1992, pp. 347–351). Again, "more of the same" does not make a change.[8] As Einstein is often credited with saying, "The definition of insanity is doing the same thing over and over again but expecting different results."

Kottler's genuinely angry outburst, described in Chapter 15, cut through his client's disingenuousness.[9] Hillary and Brad Keeney's (Chapter 13) unique improvisations awakened the session, opening new ways of healing for their client. Both Karin Schlanger (Chapter 17) and Terry Soo-Hoo (Chapter 19) surprised and delighted their clients by encouraging them to act flirtatiously with their spouses to disrupt marital quarreling.

Paul Watzlawick (1978) emphasized the importance of impactful language, including the use of phrasings that engage our brains. The unexpected creates curiosity and sets the mind searching (Rossi & Rossi, 2014; Hill & Rossi, 2017). Steve de Shazer and Elam Nunnally (1991, pp. 263–264) at the Brief Family Therapy Center (Milwaukee) reported de Shazer saying to a couple who presented a puzzling dilemma: "You've got a problem … In short, we don't know what the f--- you are going to do. I suggest that you think about what I just said, and decide what actions you are going to take." One of us (MFH) has gotten a lot of good therapeutic mileage when counseling people with problematic substance use by quoting the slogan "Reality is for people who can't handle drugs," rather than the usual shaming "Drugs are for people who can't handle reality" – the former creates for listeners a *"You Said What?"* moment that catches their ears and may lead into a nuanced discussion about distinctions between substance use and abuse. Similarly, Socrates may have said that "The unexamined life is not worth living," but another "reversed" line that has helped to engage many clients in a discussion about their problems and therapy goals is "The unlived life is worth examining."

Humor. In several of the examples in this volume, one can imagine the twinkle in the therapists' eyes as a *You Said What?* message was conveyed. Humor often involves surprise and the release of tension, producing mirth and laughter (see Hurley, Dennett, & Adams, 2011). "It is ever a source of fresh amazement when the unconscious processes express weighty and troublesome problems in a short-hand which has in it an element of levity" said Milton Erickson (1940/1980, p. 186). Frank Farrelly and Scott Matthews (2001, p. 534) echoed: "Laughter is the sound of victory."

Victor Frankl (1991, p. 102) advised that paradoxical interventions be promulgated "with tongue in cheek." Carl Whitaker (1975) emphasized the normalizing use of absurdity in the psychotherapy of aggression. In an episode, for example, that engenders *You Said What?* reactions from many readers, Whitaker recounted (1975, p. 5) that when a patient threatened to harm him, Whitaker called a colleague (John Warkentin) into the session with the patient. When the colleague heard the patient's threat he exclaimed, "I don't blame you a bit. I've often wanted to kill Whitaker myself!"

"Humorous interventions in therapy include an element of surprise, of the unexpected. A humorous definition, explanation, or directive ... gives strength, drama, and impact to an intervention" (Madanes, 2006a, p. 259). A well-timed joke or *bon mot* can produce a *You Said What?* reaction, as many listeners had when they heard that a grieving taxi driver had been told the one about another driver who got stopped by a cop and, when the police officer said that he wouldn't get a ticket if he had a good story, the cabbie replied (switching rejection to escape) "My wife ran off with a cop. When I saw you, I got scared you were him, and that you were bringing her back!" (see Hoyt & Ritterman, 2012, p. 7). Steve Andreas, a well-known NLP practitioner, generated a big *You Said What?* audience chuckle when he suggested telling someone who was hypochondriacal or otherwise uncomfortable with normal bodily sensations about the very straight-laced young man who said, when he got sexually aroused and had an erection, "My mother always told me that if I looked at a naked woman I'd turn to stone, and now it's starting to happen" (Hoyt & Andreas, 2015, p. 20).[10]

Context. Interventions that produce *You Said What?* reactions reorganize relationships, change power dynamics, and shift meanings. As Carlos Sluzki (1998, p. 163) wrote:

> By the way in which we manage the therapeutic dialogue, we generate in and with our clients (or at least we plant the seed along the way for) a series of possible options, a set of potential strange attractors, that contribute to the possibility that the presenting stories will be reconfigured around those new organizing principles as stories that are distinctly and qualitatively different, that have a "better form."

The parents in Bertolino's case (Chapter 3) said they got "a different education" as they provided their wayward son with "a different education";

Goldfield encouraged an anorectic girl and obese father to change roles in Chapter 8; Hoyt's post-stroke client in Chapter 10 became more empowered when the therapist literally went "one down" on to the floor and asked the client for coaching; Keeney and Keeney's client in Chapter 13 got excited by their improvisations and began to imagine himself and his skin condition in new and more encouraging ways. In Chapter 16, Ritterman noted that while Milton Erickson is perhaps best known for inducing hypnosis, symptoms can be thought of as socially induced trances and much of Erickson's (and Ritterman's) work involves assisting people to break bad spells and wake up from dysfunctional trances. Indeed, Clara Solís demonstrated this in Chapter 18 when the mother and daughter changed their image of the daughter and began to interact differently when she helped them discover Frida Kahlo.[11]

Acceptability. A *You Said What?* intervention facilitates reframing[12] and client acceptance by emphasizing clients' strengths and resources that fit the desired outcome (motivation) and preferred view of self/others (Eron & Lund, 1996).[13] Andy Austin (Chapter 2) aided a woman to stop participating in cocaine parties by appealing to her protective maternal instincts; Bob Bertolino (Chapter 3) helped his clients feel that they were better parenting their teenage son; Jim Duvall's client (Chapter 6) was willing to risk the anxiety of exposure to a group because she was able to see it as an avenue to becoming a better mother; Douglas Flemons (Chapter 7) used carefully chosen language to help his client *en*counter (rather than resist) bodily functions; Esther Krohner (Chapter 17) reconceptualizing her teenage client's violent imagery as essentially a form of protectiveness appealed to his motivation to become more loving toward his parents; and Solís and Vargas in Chapter 18 guided mother and daughter to have experiences that allowed them to envision a more hopeful future; and Terry Soo-Hoo facilitated his client's finding a culturally compatible solution.

Memorable. *You Said What?* interventions stick in the mind. We all can probably recall having heard someone begin a story by saying, "Did you hear about ...?" *You Said What?* moments stay with us because their accuracy and wit open doors.[14]

The Inspiration of Creative Therapists

There was a time, especially in the 1970s and 80s, when many water-cooler and late-night-in-the-lounge therapy discussions began with "Did you hear about what Milton Erickson (or Carl Whitaker, Sal Minuchin, Harry Goolishian, or another luminary) said ...?" In our invitation to potential contributors (Chapter 1), Erickson was the therapist in the cases of Jesus in the carpenter shop, the bedwetter being directed to pee into his bed, and the taunting of a prideful stroke victim to provoke him to take action (see Haley, 1973); Whitaker was the therapist deliberately infuriating the teenage girl in the E.R. to reject self-harm by talking about who would get her possessions and how long it would take for her ex-boyfriend to resume dating (reported in Hoyt,

2017, pp. 308-309). A transcript of Harry Goolishian's charmingly uncommon way of working with a distraught client who wanted to donate his body to medical science after poisoning himself is provided by Bobele in Chapter 4.

To tell just one more *You Said What?* story, back in 1980 I (MFH) attended a workshop at the Berkeley Family Institute to see Salvador Minuchin work. In a demonstration interview with an anorectic family, the teenage girl was seated between her parents and they were each giving her contradictory, double-binding messages. Minuchin said to the girl, "Your father has one of your ears and your mother has your other ear, but you still have your own brain – so you can decide." The father, resistant and rude, turned to Minuchin and said, "Who says you know anything?'" Minuchin looked compassionately at him and his family, then gestured toward the audience (a couple hundred people) and replied, "I'm trying to help your daughter – and I can assure you, they came to hear me."

The creative interventions appearing in this volume may not all be astounding and prototypal, but all the authors, in their own extraordinary ways, continue the tradition of creatively and disruptively thinking "outside the box" of conventional therapy in those challenging situations when it might be tempting to become rote and conservative. As Steve de Shazer (in Hoyt, 1996/2001, pp. 159–161) commented, the goal is not to be especially clever or sensationalistic but, rather, to evoke client resources.

Stanley Messer and Seth Warren (1995) discern four different "visions of reality" that influence therapists: the romantic, the comic, the ironic, and the tragic. Wherever you're coming from, it sure helps to have that twinkle in your eye, to be playful and to have a sense of humor.

Further Considerations

Timing, context, and cultural sensitivity are paramount. In Chapter 9 Shelley Green was smart to work with, not against, her clients' (unusual) beliefs and lifestyle. Haley (1984) and others have warned against prescribing an ordeal that is dangerous, immoral, or illegal. All interventions should be consistent with general ethical principles, especially those of beneficence and non-maleficence (Foreman, 1990).

Cloé Madanes (1990, pp. 213–214) agreed that clinicians craft stories that they hope will positively influence their clients:

> [F]amily members come to the therapy with one view of the obstacles that they find overwhelming. The therapist transforms these obstacles into new difficulties that can be resolved ... With reframing, magic is introduced ... [R]eframing introduces to the family meaning, drama, and the possibility of being someone else, of relating and living in ways that have gone unsuspected. The truth of the reframing depends on its own persuasive powers, on the skill of the magic. Every good therapy tells the truth and every bad therapy lies. Truth in therapy is to make the client experience

an illusion; manipulation and lies mean to be unable to accomplish that trickery. Therapy has its own ethic, one in which truth and falsehood are secondary concepts.

In Chapter 4, I (MB) mentioned that following the publication of Bobele (1987), a critique from a social worker and a psychologist/lawyer (Woody & Woody, 1988) was published in *JMFT*. These authors took issue with my approach in the cases, arguing that my colleagues and I had ignored "the therapist's responsibility to prevent the dangerous behavior" (p. 133). They went on to outline important features of public policy and pointed out how, in both cases, they believed that we had blatantly ignored public policy, endangered our clients, and failed in our duty to warn. However, they offered no alternative suggestions about how the cases should have been handled. In John Weakland's (1988, p. 205) letter to the editor, he speculated that "though apparently it [the Woodys' method] would involve commonsensical and conventional steps" he went on to caution: "While such courses are almost always safest for the *therapist,* in many instances there is reason to think they will not minimize danger to the client and others involved. (If otherwise, these cases would not pose such difficult problems in the first place.)" That was exactly the point. Conventional steps had already been attempted and failed, and the problematic behavior was apparently escalating. There were two important footnotes in the original article that may have been overlooked by the Woodys: First, "It is difficult to convey in print the affective tone, pacing, and careful attention to the client's body language that [I] attended to while delivering [these interventions]" (p. 239). The second important footnote, that is relevant as we consider the various *You Said What?* moments described in this volume, was "Unfortunately, all too many therapists mistake nonsensical and weird interventions with good systemic therapy. ... A grave error is committed when a therapist believes that the intervention is what should be weird, unexpected or uncommonsensical" (p. 239).

Although some might be tempted to emulate the techniques described in this book, we caution against directly copying the interventions. We hope that you will, instead, be inspired by their inventiveness.[15] One critical aspect of a *You Said What?* intervention is customizing the message, task, or directive to be congruent with the unique values, language, customs, and context of both the therapist and the client. I (MB) once again recall the wisdom of my mentor, Harry Goolishian, who, paraphrasing Heraclitus ("No one ever steps in the same river twice"), advised that "A good intervention is like a kitchen match – it only works once. "

An Invitation: You'll Say What?

We hope that the *You Said What?* moments you have read about here will inspire you to think about new ways you might work. Next time you or your client are stuck, what might you do to stretch beyond your usual repertoires? How will you disrupt unsuccessful attempted solutions and evoke energy and new perspectives? *You'll say WHAT?*

Notes

1 To use Piaget's (1977) learning theory terminology, they require *accommodation*, not just *assimilation*. And, as Gary Saul Morson (1994, p. 24) said in his book *Narrative and Freedom*, "For creativity to be real, it must be a genuine *process* of undetermined becoming: it cannot be the mere unfolding of an already completely determined sequence of steps to a ready-made conclusion."

2 "He that has eyes to see and ears to hear may convince himself that no mortal can keep a secret. If his lips are silent, he chatters with his fingertips; betrayal oozes out of him at every pore. And thus the task of making conscious the most hidden recesses of the mind is one which is quite possible to accomplish" – Sigmund Freud (1905/1953, pp. 77–78).

3 Loriedo and Vella (1992, pp. 146–148) provide a catalogue of counterparadoxical injunctions, beginning with Frankl's *paradoxical intention*.

4 "We do not see things as they are. We see things as we are" – Anaïs Nin (1989, p. 124).

5 "Empathy is the capacity to take up the perspective of another person, that is, to see things as that person sees them and to feel what that person feels. It is conceptualized metaphorically as the capacity to project your consciousness into other people, so that you can experience *what* they experience, the *way* they experience it" – Lakoff & Johnson (1999, p. 309).

6 "You are using his own words to alter the patient's access to his various frames of reference" (Erickson & Rossi, 1981, p. 255).

7 Long ago, I (MFH) was a predoctoral intern with Carl Whitaker (who was the main inspiration for Keith's symbolic experiential approach). Trainees would sometimes try to imitate Whitaker's famous, seemingly unpredictable and zany style but without the connection, caring, and deep resonance that Whitaker had (and Keith has). Their remarks usually came across as rude and bizarre, not therapeutic. Whitaker once said to me (MFH, personal communication, 1974): "Love is the anesthesia that allows the surgery to be successful." Frank Farrelly, the main developer of Provocative Therapy (see Farrelly & Brandsma, 1974), had a way of looking at clients, as he mocked their foolishness, that said that he really cared about them. Along related lines, when Jay Haley (quoted in Davis, 2011, p. 26) was asked, "If you could teach students only one thing, what would it be?' he answered without hesitation: "Love. I'd teach them to love their clients. Everything else falls into place once a therapist loves their clients." One time (reported in Hoyt, 2017, pp. 185–186), deeply connected to a grieving couple, I was inspired to take the unusual action of sending a bottle of champagne to their dinner table to acknowledge their loss and support their recovery.

8 Thus, Bill O'Hanlon (1999) succinctly advised, "Do one thing different."

9 This episode occurred within the context of Kottler's caring and compassion. Although the expression of therapist anger sometimes can be helpful (see Winnicott, 1949), not all angry outbursts, of course, are *You Said What?* therapeutic moments.

Hoyt (2003), for example, reports an instance wherein his frustration and irritable abruptness drove a client away without benefit.

10   As Farrelly and Brandsma (1974, pp. 97–98) observed: "[A] joke can be seen as consisting of two parts, the setting up of a context and a punch line. Within an established context (ground) the punch line has as one of its main effects the reversing of the context very abruptly and bringing new elements into the figure … With the punch line the rules of reality have become temporarily jumbled … Uncertainty can be very beneficial when it causes a person to examine his behavior, attitude, or construct of reality more carefully or from a different vantage point." Long ago, Freud (1928/1961) noted that humor can say, in effect, that a situation is serious but there are other ways to look at it that might even give one some pleasure.

11   Jay Haley (Haley & Richeport-Haley, 2003) once reported that when other therapeutic gambits had failed, he put a mother in charge by directing her to pay money to two young brothers to stop their misbehavior. (He did *What?!*) The intervention was successful: the family hierarchy and interactional dynamics shifted and the boys' bad behavior desisted. Cloé Madanes (2006b, p. 115) similarly reports a case in which a mother was paid to not hit her 10-year-old son; after several months, relationships realigned, payment was discontinued, and the child was not abused again. Madanes, Keim, and Smelser (1995) also describe a dramatic, step-by-step process that restructures hierarchy in which violent/abusive men are required to humble themselves before the victim and family by kneeling, acknowledging their wrongdoings, and apologizing.

12   "To reframe, then, means to change the conceptual and/or emotional setting or viewpoint in relation to which a situation is experienced and to place it in another frame which fits the 'facts' of the same concrete situation equally well or even better, and thereby changes its entire meaning" (Watzlawick et al., 1974, p. 95). As Fisch and Schlanger (1999, p. 19) have written, "In order to encourage people to depart from their customary efforts, it is no simple matter of telling them what different tack they should take … [P]eople persist in what they do because they regard it as the only reasonable thing to do, the only correct thing. Simply to suggest something very different is to challenge their reality. Thus, any new tack or direction needs to be framed, packaged if you will, in an explanation that is likely to be palatable to the client." Providing a convincing "morale restoring" rationale is generally part of healing and persuasion (Frank & Frank, 1991).

13   In 1946 (pp. 66–70), Franz Alexander and Thomas French cited the example, from Victor Hugo's *Les Misérables*, of the convicted thief, Jean Valjean, switching from sinner to saint when the bishop dramatically and unexpectedly forgave him for stealing the silver candlesticks. It was a *"You Said What?* moment for the thief – and for many readers. This "single session therapy" conversion, which Alexander and French termed a "corrective emotional experience," was triggered by the bishop's forgiveness, which disconfirmed Jean Valjean's expectations and awakened reminders of his own goodness (see Hoyt, 2017, p. 232).

14   "Humor is the ultimate shorthand" – Mort Sahl (1976, p. 23).

15   "When someone points to the sky, look at the moon – not the finger" – Zen saying.

References

Alexander, F., & French, T.M. (1946). *Psychoanalytic therapy: Theory and applications.* New York: Ronald Press.

Ansbacher, H.L., & Ansbacher, R.R. (Eds.). (1956). *The individual psychology of Alfred Adler.* New York: Basic Books.

Bobele, M. (1987). Therapeutic interventions in life-threatening situations. *Journal of Marriage and Family Therapy, 13*(3), 225–239.

Budman, S.H., Hoyt, M.F., & Friedman, S. (Eds.). (1992). *The first session in brief therapy.* New York: Guilford Press.

Davis, S. (2011, November/December). Models or therapists: Power from a common factors perspective. *Family Therapy Magazine, 10*(6), 26–28.

de Shazer, S. (1988). *Clues: Investigating solutions in brief therapy.* New York: Norton.

de Shazer, S, & Nunnally, E. (1991). The mysterious affair of paradoxes and loops. In G.R. Weeks (Ed.). *Promoting change through paradoxical therapy* (rev. ed., pp. 252–270). New York: Brunner/Mazel.

Erickson, M.H. (1980). The translation of the automatic writing of one hypnotic subject by another in a trance-like dissociated state. In *Collected papers* (Vol. 3; E.L. Rossi, Ed.). New York: Irvington. (Work originally published 1940.)

Erickson, M.H., & Rossi, E.L. (1981). *Experiencing hypnosis.* New York: Irvington.

Eron, J.B., & Lund, T.W. (1996). *Narrative solutions in brief therapy.* New York: Guilford Press.

Farrelly, F., & Brandsma, J. (1974). *Provocative therapy.* Capitola, CA: Meta Publications.

Farrelly, F., & Matthews, S. (2001). Provocative therapy. In R.J. Corsini (Ed.). *Handbook of innovative therapy* (2nd ed.; pp. 523–534). New York: Wiley.

Fisch, R. L., & Schlanger, K. (1999). *Brief therapy with intimidating cases: Changing the unchangeable.* San Francisco: Jossey-Bass.

Foreman, D.M. (1990). The ethical use of paradoxical interventions in psychotherapy. *Journal of Medical Ethics, 16*, 200–205.

Frank, J. D., & Frank, J. B. (1991). *Healing and persuasion: A comparitive study of psychtherapy* (3rd ed.). Baltimore, MD: Johns Hopkins University Press.

Frankl, V. (1991). Paradoxical intention. In G.R. Weeks (Ed.). *Promoting change through paradoxical therapy* (pp. 99–110). New York: Brunner/Mazel.

Fraser, J.S., & Solovey, A.D. (2007). *Second-order change in psychotherapy: The golden thread that unifies effective treatments.* Washington, DC: APA Books.

Freud, S. (1953). Fragment of an analysis of a case of hysteria. In *Standard edition of the complete psychological works of Sigmund Freud* (Vol. 7, pp. 1–122). London: Hogarth Press. (Work originally published 1905.)

Freud, S. (1961). Humour. *In Standard edition of the complete psychological works of Sigmund Freud* (Vol. 21, pp. 159–166). London: Hogarth Press. (Work originally published 1928)

Haley, J. (1973). *Uncommon therapy: The psychiatric techniques of Milton H. Erickson, M.D.* New York: Norton.

Haley, J. (1984). *Ordeal therapy: Unusual ways to change behavior.* San Francisco: Jossey-Bass.

Haley, J., & Richeport-Haley, M. (2003). Changing a violent family. In *The art of strategic therapy* (pp. 79–95). New York: Brunner-Routledge.

Hill, R., & Rossi, E.L. (2017). *The practitioner's guide to mirroring hands.* Williston, VT: Crown House Publishing.

Hoffman, L. (1990). Constructing realities: An art of lenses. *Family Process, 29*, 1–12.

Hoyt, M.F. (2000). *Some stories are better than others: Doing what works in brief therapy and managed care.* New York: Brunner/Mazel.

Hoyt, M.F. (2001). Solution building and language game: A conversation with Steve de Shazer (and some after words with Insoo Kim Berg). In M.F. Hoyt (Int.), *Interviews with brief therapy experts* (pp. 158–183). New York: Brunner-Routledge. (Work originally published 1996)

Hoyt, M.F. (2003). I was blind at the time. In J.A. Kottler & J. Carlson (Eds.). *Bad therapy: Master therapists share their worst failures* (pp. 157–164). New York: Brunner-Routledge.

Hoyt, M.F. (2017). *Brief therapy and beyond: Stories, language, love, hope, and time.* New York: Routledge.

Hoyt, M.F., & Andreas, S. (2015). Humor in brief therapy: A dialogue – Part I. *Journal of Systemic Therapies, 34*(1), 13–24.

Hoyt, M.F., & Ritterman, M. (2012). Brief therapy in a taxi. *Milton H. Erickson Foundation Newsletter, 32*(2), 7.

Hurley, M.M., Dennett, D.C., & Adams, Jr., R.B. (2011). *Inside jokes: Using humor to reverse-engineer the mind.* Cambridge, MA: MIT Press.

Lakoff, G., & Johnson, M. (1999). *Philosophy in the flesh: The embodied mind and its challenge to Western thought.* New York: Basic Books.

Levin, C., Shapiro, F., & Weakland, J.H. (1996). When the past is present: A conversation about EMDR and the MRI interactional approach. In M.F. Hoyt (Ed.). *Constructive therapies 2* (pp. 197–210). New York: Guilford Press.

Linehan, M.M. (1993). *Cognitive-behavioral treatment of borderline personality disorder.* New York: Guilford Press.

Loriedo, C., & Vella, G. (1992). *Paradox and the family system.* New York: Brunner/Mazel.

Madanes, C. (1990). *Sex, love, and violence: Strategies for transformation.* New York: Norton.

Madanes, C. (2006a). "Hey, did you hear the one about …" In *The therapist as humanist, social activist, and systemic thinker … and other selected papers* (pp. 248–260). Phoenix, AZ: Zeig, Tucker, & Theisen.

Madanes, C. (2006b). Money and the family. In *The therapist as humanist, social activist, and systemic thinker … and other selected papers* (pp. 97–117). Phoenix, AZ: Zeig, Tucker, & Theisen.

Madanes, C., Keim, J.P., & Smelser, D. (1995). *The violence of men: New techniques for working with abusive families: A therapy of social action.* San Francisco: Jossey-Bass.

Messer, S.B., & Warren, C.S. (1995). *Models of brief psychodynamic therapy: A comparative approach.* New York: Guilford Press.

Morson, G.S. (1994). *Narrative and freedom: The shadows of time.* New Haven, CT: Yale University Press.

Nin, A. (1989). *Seduction of the minotaur.* Athens, OH: Swallow Press/Ohio University Press.

O'Hanlon, W.H. (1999). *Do one thing different: And other uncommonly sensible solutions to life's persistent problems.* New York: William Morrow.

Piaget, J. (1977). *The essential Piaget: An interpretive reference and guide* (H.E. Gruber & J.J. Vonéche, Eds.). New York: Basic Books.

Rossi, K., & Rossi, E.L. (2014). Opening the heart and mind with single session psychotherapy and therapeutic hypnosis: A final meeting with Milton H. Erickson M.D. – Part 1. In M.F. Hoyt & M. Talmon (Eds.). *Capturing the moment: Single session therapy and walk-in services* (pp. 233–253). Bethel, CT: Crown House Publishing.

Rowa, K., Antony, M. M., & Swinson, R. P. (2007). Exposure and response prevention. In M. M. Antony, C. Purdon, & L. J. Summerfeldt (Eds.), *Psychological treatment of obsessive-compulsive disorder: Fundamentals and beyond* (pp. 79–109). Washington, DC: American Psychological Association.

Sahl, M. (1976). *Heartland.* New York: Harcourt Brace Jovanovich.

Sluzki, C.E. (1998). Strange attractors and the transformation of narratives in family therapy. In M.F. Hoyt (Ed.), *The handbook of constructive therapies* (pp. 159–179). San Francisco: Jossey-Bass.

Watzlawick, P. (1978). *The language of change: Elements of therapeutic communication.* New York: Norton.

Watzlawick, P., Weakland, J.H., & Fisch, R. (1974). *Change: Principles of problem formation and problem resolution.* New York: Norton.

Weakland, J. H. (1988). Weakland on the Woodys-Bobele exchange. *Journal of Marital and Family Therapy, 14*(2), 205.

Whitaker, C.A. (1975). Psychotherapy of the absurd: With a special emphasis on the psychotherapy of aggression. *Family Process, 14*, 1–16.

Winnicott, D.W. (1949). Hate in the countertransference. *International Journal of Psychoanalysis, 30*, 69–74.

Woody, J. D., & Woody, R. H. (1988). Public policy in life-threatening situations: A response to Bobele. *Journal of Marital and Family Therapy, 14*(2), 133–137.

Index

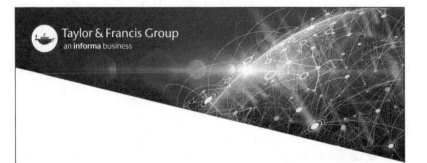